THE
IMAGE OF AMERICA
IN
MAZZINI'S WRITINGS

JOSEPH ROSSI

MADISON, WISCONSIN
THE UNIVERSITY OF WISCONSIN PRESS · 1954

Published by
The University of Wisconsin Press
811 State Street, Madison 5, Wisconsin

Copyright, Canada, 1954. Distributed in Canada by Burns
& MacEachern, Toronto. Printed in the Netherlands by
N. V. Drukkerij G. J. Thieme, Nijmegen. Library of Congress
Catalogue Card Number 54–6743.

FOREWORD

EARLY STUDENTS of Mazzini were under the impression that the great Italian revolutionist ignored the United States in his political thinking and global schemes. Both Bolton King and Gaetano Salvemini asserted, early in the century, that he did not take into much account the United States and that in his mind humanity was equated to the European countries to whom the rest of the world, divided into spheres of influence, was assigned for the performance of a civilizing mission. But as more of Mazzini's writings came to light, it became apparent that this impression was not quite correct in its bearing on America. In the early twenties Alessandro Luzio, an eminent Mazzini scholar, called attention to the numerous contacts Mazzini had with the United States that were, and in the main still are, not well known.

The present monograph is a contribution toward the study of these contacts. As its title implies, it is limited to an investigation of only those connections which are mentioned in Mazzini's works. American sources—periodical literature, daily press, etc.—have been used only to illustrate those contacts to which Mazzini refers in his writings and in which we may presume he was interested. No attempt has been made to survey systematically American public opinion for a story of the fortunes of Mazzinianism in America—which can very well be the subject of a separate study. Nor has any attempt been made to determine what influence, if any, Mazzini exerted on American liberal thinkers. This writer hopes that some scholar fully conversant with the history of American liberal thought may deem the subject worthy of investigation.

The primary source on which this study has been based is the National Edition of Mazzini's *Scritti editi ed inediti*, recently

v

brought to completion in one hundred volumes. All references
are given from this edition. Quotations from Mazzini's English
writings are given in the original, and the stylistic and idiomatic
peculiarities of Mazzini's English are preserved; those from his
Italian or French writings are given in this writer's translation. It
was not considered necessary to indicate in each case the language
of the original.

The author is indebted to numerous scholars in the field, and
his indebtedness is scrupulously indicated in the notes. He feels,
however, that a special acknowledgment is due to three American
scholars whose works threw badly needed light on some phases
of his investigation: to Professor H. R. Marraro, for his *American
Opinion on the Unification of Italy*; to Dr. L. F. Stock, for his
edition of consular and diplomatic dispatches and reports of American representatives at the papal court; and to Professor M. E.
Curti for his paper on "Young America."

The author takes pleasure in expressing his gratitude to those
who helped him in the preparation of this study: to the Research
Committee of the Graduate School of the University of Wisconsin
which assigned a grant, from special funds voted by the State
Legislature, to initiate this study; to Mr. Guido Capponi, a Graduate Assistant in Italian at the University of Wisconsin, who
located and copied a number of references in New Orleans newspapers; to Mr. Lester G. Wells, Curator of the Gerrit Smith
Miller Collection at the Syracuse University Library, who called
his attention to, and supplied a transcript of, an unpublished letter
of Gerrit Smith to Mazzini; to the staffs of the Wisconsin Historical Library and the Library of the University of Wisconsin for
their assistance and unfailing courtesy; and to his wife, who
patiently and skilfully typed the various drafts of this monograph.

Madison, Wisconsin   JOSEPH ROSSI
December, 1953

CONTENTS

Chapter I

EARLY NOTIONS OF AMERICA

THE AMERICAN Revolution stirred considerable interest among eighteenth century Italian liberal thinkers, who looked upon it not as the rebellion of a group of colonies against the mother country but as the beginning of a movement of liberation from tyranny that would embrace all humankind. To a great extent, this conception was fostered by the language of the Declaration of Independence, which expressed ideas typical of the Illuministic philosophy, and by the skillful propaganda of Benjamin Franklin, who, already famous in Europe as a natural philosopher, during his stay in Paris confirmed the notion of European liberals that he, so simple in manners, so wise, so dignified, was the prototype of American republicans.

In the eyes of those liberals the American Revolutionary War acquired great importance for the effect it would have on the rest of the world. It would decide the destiny of humanity, according to one writer; it would make that period memorable for centuries to come, according to another. In establishing free institutions the Americans would prove, and, indeed, had the duty to prove, that their free form of government was superior to all others. America would become the ideal fatherland of all liberals, a beacon to all people of the earth, "the happy corner of the earth where good faith, liberty, equality, and virtue have taken refuge," as one of them put it.

Curiously mixed with this exemplary role assigned to America was the idea of a retributive justice to be eventually meted out by an aroused and powerful America to the European imperial powers—England, France, and Spain—for the cruel exploitation colonies on the new continent had suffered at the hands of the mother countries. Filangieri, Genovesi, Galiani, all make, in

I

various forms, the forecast of a future conquest of Europe by America and the establishment of American colonies in Europe. Even before the Revolution, Galiani expressed the opinion that the center of what is now called Western civilization would shift westward to America, since the progress of civilization had always followed the course of the sun; and later he jokingly advised his Parisian friend Madame d'Épinay to buy her new home not at the Chaussée-d'Antin but in Philadelphia.

The idea of a palingenesis of civilization in America, and of the salvation of the Old World by the New by example or by conquest, was especially popular in Italian Freemasons' circles, and through them reached the most unexpected corners of the country. In 1783, the village of Castelmonardo in Calabria was destroyed by an earthquake. The Serra family, leading landowners of the place and member of the Freemasonry, had the town rebuilt at their expense and renamed Filadelfia not only because of the etymological meaning of the name but also because that was the name of the capital of the United States.[1]

It is well known that in his early youth Mazzini was a member of that offshoot of Freemasonry, the Carbonari Society. It is likely that traces of the mystical, symbolic idea of the New World still existed among the Carbonari and were absorbed by Mazzini, first in the family circle and later at lodge meetings. The fact that in his early youth Mazzini did show a significant, though by no means overwhelming, interest in America is revealed by his *Zibaldoni* (notebooks), which have been preserved, in which he jotted notes on the founding fathers—Washington, Samuel Adams, "the American Cato," John Adams, Franklin—on the slave trade, the conditions of the slaves, and on other American topics.[2]

It is true, however, that when Mazzini initiated his lifelong work of republican propaganda his knowledge of American life and culture was not very extensive. The references found in his early published works, besides some laudatory commonplaces on Washington and Franklin, show only some acquaintance with the works of James Fenimore Cooper. The American novelist is said by Mazzini to be, together with Scott, Van-der-Velde, and Zschokke, one of the writers who made the historical novel "a citizen of Europe";[3] his story *The Prairie* had suggested one of the characters in Varese's *La Fidanzata Ligure* (*1* : 28). Since Cooper at that time had already achieved considerable popularity in Italy,[4] Mazzini's acquaintance with his novels can hardly be taken as an indication of extensive knowledge of America.

Even when after years of residence in England Mazzini had achieved great ease in the use of the English language, his knowledge of American literature remained scanty. Besides Cooper, the only American writers he mentioned were Emerson, whom he admired with some reservations, Theodore Parker, Harriet Beecher Stowe, and O. W. Holmes.[5] No mention is found in his published works of writers already well known in Europe such as Irving, Poe, Thoreau, Whitman, Longfellow, unless some of them are referred to in the cryptic statement made in a note to a friend in 1857 to the effect that "American poetry is sickening" (60 : 182). Of course, this lack of interest may have been due to the well known fact that early in life Mazzini sacrificed literature to political evangelism and revolutionary action. The polemical contingencies of his republican propaganda led his attention to another and, to him, more important aspect of American culture—the political.

The Italian aspirations after liberty and independence aroused by the Napoleonic period were disregarded by the Congress of Vienna. The restoration of the *status quo* made the peninsula a political powder keg. Secret political societies, especially the *Carbonari* (charcoal-makers), spread rapidly throughout the country, and revolutionary movements followed shortly—in Naples in 1820–21, in Piedmont in 1821, in the Papal States and the neighboring duchies of Parma and Modena in 1831. All those rebellions succeeded with unbelievable ease in overthrowing local regimes, but they were then put down with equal ease by the Austrian military power.

Giuseppe Mazzini was born on June 22, 1805, in Genoa, a city with a long and glorious republican past, which was arbitrarily handed over to the Sardinian king by the Congress of Vienna. Mazzini, a young lawyer and promising literary critic, joined the *Carbonari* and rose quickly to the rank of organizer, but he soon grew dissatisfied with their ritualism and the vagueness of their political aims. When he was arrested because of his political activities and held in the fortress of Savona for several months he employed that enforced leisure for a serious consideration of ways, means, and prospects of the *Carbonari* and reached the conclusion that a new and different society should be organized to take up the work of political regeneration of the country. On his release from prison early in 1831, he went to France to escape the restrictions imposed on him by the Sardinian police, and shortly after he founded that new society—Young Italy.

When Mazzini went to France the era of good feelings between the July Monarchy and the Republican party still prevailed. The government of Louis Philippe had not yet openly repudiated the republican program of democratic reforms at home and revolutionary expansionism abroad. In that atmosphere vibrant with republican hopes, aspirations, dreams, and schemes, Mazzini drew the broad outline of his political philosophy which in later years was elaborated and expanded but never modified substantially and which in its basic points shows clearly the influence of French republican thought.[6] The ideas which he expressed in 1832 in his letter to the Swiss historian Sismondi—"unitarian" republican system with large local autonomy, popular sovereignty, or "government of the country by the country," legislative action to raise the standard of living of the lower classes, abolition of all special privileges, progressive taxation, freedom of the press, freedom of association, universal elementary education, trial by jury, etc. (*3* : 18)—are similar to the ideas expounded by Leroux, Trélat, Arago, Raspail, Dornès, and other left-wing republicans at that very time.[7] The very name of the political association he founded, Young Italy, may have been suggested to him by the name of a newspaper, *Jeune France*, which had been published in Paris for a few months in 1829.

But if Mazzini was a disciple of the French republicans, he was not a very docile one. He rejected their basic assumption that man has some natural, inalienable rights. Keeping in mind the peculiar problems of Italy, divided as it was into several small states each oppressed and exploited by some foreign or domestic tyrant, he realized that the theory of individual rights was not the lever he needed to move the Italians to act for the liberty and unification of their country. If single individuals, communities, or classes obtained the enjoyment of their own rights, they would have no motivation for the possible sacrifice of life and substance which the task of Italian redemption required. This consideration led Mazzini to reverse the basis of the current liberal political thought and to set *duty* as the corner stone of his political edifice.

Life, he asserted, is a mission; life is the fulfillment of a duty for individuals as well as communities. The individual must be free because only thus can he develop fully his potentialities and make his best contribution to the nation; and the nation in return has the duty to place the citizen in the conditions which will permit the fulfillment of his social duties and, hence, permit the enjoyment of his rights. The same principle he applied to nations, "the individuals of humanity." Each country has a mission, a task for which it is peculiarly fitted by geographical, cultural, historical factors, and it must be free and independent in order to fulfill its mission for the benefit of humanity; and humanity joined in a federation of free and independent nations has in return the duty to put each member nation in the best condition to perform that task necessary for the fulfillment of humanity's own mission, the gradual ascension of all humankind in accordance with the law of progress, which is the law of God. Mazzini's social fabric was thus woven not out of mutually limiting rights but out of reciprocally supplementing duties. For him a right existed only where there was a duty to perform. Thus Mazzini denied the Irish the right to a separate nation, because he could not perceive a "mission" for them distinct from that of the British nationality.

From this standpoint, Mazzini examined contemporary French republican thought and found it faulty, because it was dominated by the exclusive principle of rights—e.g., the rights of the community demanded by the left-wing group, which was ready to sacrifice liberty to equality and which was concerned only, as he later put it, "in organizing the kitchen of Humanity" (44 : 41) and the rights of the individual demanded by the right-wing group—the "American" school—which stifled the principle of association under the omnipotence of the individual, established distrust in the civil organization, and enthroned selfish interests, materialism, and contradiction (6 : 348–49).

It was especially against the American school that Mazzini turned his polemical attacks, because it was more influential and enjoyed more prestige with his fellow exiles from Italy. This faction, led first by Lafayette, then by Armand Carrel, took the American constitution as its ideal, hence its name, and stood for the well-behaved, conservative republic opposed to all radicalism, such as progressive taxation, social reforms, and the like. It advocated the sort of republicanism that could be accepted by a constitutional monarchist, and was in fact ostensibly accepted by Louis Philippe himself. Lafayette reported to his constituency that before he lent his support to the monarchy during the July revolution he had an interview with the Duke of Orléans in which he informed the prince, later King Louis Philippe, that he was a republican and that he considered the Constitution of the United States the most perfect ever made. To which the prince replied that, having spent two years in America himself, he was bound to agree with him completely.[8] When radicalism reared its threatening head shortly afterwards, Lafayette disassociated himself with that brand of republicanism, protesting that, as a friend of Washington, Franklin, and Jefferson, he was not tempted to change parish for the patronage of Robespierre, Saint-Just, and Marat.[9] The radicals, on the other hand, sneered at the American model: the writers of the *Moniteur républicain*, in the style of their future comrades of the Cominform, defined the United States as a "ridiculous, aristocratic republic of money grabbers."[10]

Mazzini opposed the American school not only for the theoretical reason mentioned, namely, the excessive, exclusive rule assigned to individual rights, but also for some practical reasons. He resented the claim of exclusive French leadership of the republican revolution and abhorred the principle of federation on the American and Swiss model urged by them on other countries outside France. The French, as the direct heirs to the principles of 1789 suppressed by the Congress of Vienna, maintained that it was the role of their country to reassert them and to liberate Europe. "Revolution," said Babeuf, "is . . . our country fulfilling that mission of liberation which was assigned to it by the Providence of the Peoples."[11] This tutelage was galling to Mazzini, who noticed also that the French republicans expected to charge a fee for this liberation of the oppressed people in the form of territorial claims on the liberated lands—the Rhine provinces from Germany and Savoy from Italy.[12] The suggestion of a federal form of government for Italy and Germany was to him another evidence of French imperialism. Armand Carrel, the brilliant young editor of the *National* and acknowledged leader of the American school after the death of Lafayette whom Mazzini knew quite well, "insinuated," he said, "now and then, *federalism* for Italy, Spain, Germany, remaining unitarian for France, partly because unity there was an accomplished fact, partly because the French dominating instinct, very strong in him, showed him in that way a perpetual supremacy of his country over the weakness of the neighboring federations" (*77* : 147–48).

America [Mazzini wrote in 1833] was the arena where the first struggle took place between the principle of limited monarchy and the republic. The republic obtained there its first victory,—and that was enough for the politics of imitation to proclaim itself exclusively American. The American school, under the leadership of Lafayette, a man of rare virtue and limited ability, dominates at present the thinking of a great many republicans. In France it advocates in the columns of the *National* the bicameral system,—a patent contradiction to the principle of national sovereignty; the senate—a refuge open to the aristocracy; the *inexpensive* government—without realizing that national economy depends not on the amount of taxation, but on the manner it is employed. In Italy it advocates a federation. Why does it not advocate also the slaves, who in the American republic constitute one-seventh of the population? (*3* : 277–78)

Mazzini was rightly concerned with the dangers of this tendency to federalism, because it also dominated almost undisputed the Italian liberal thought in the thirties and forties. It was generally felt—except in Mazzini's camp—that the idea of a united Italy was a dangerous, utopian idea. The various Italian peoples had never been members of a single state since the time of the Romans, and during centuries of separate political existence they had developed their own type of civilization. The rigid frame of a single state would not be able to withstand the strain of the conflicting provincial interests, prides, loyalties, prejudices as well as a federation in which local autonomy would supply the elasticity necessary to avoid serious frictions. Furthermore, unity would be more difficult to achieve. There would be more obstacles to overcome, more vested interests to eliminate. The various ruling princes could not be expected to accept gracefully their deposition for the sake of a king of Italy or for an Italian republic. Austria would not yield peacefully her Italian provinces. There might be combined opposition to a republic from a Europe that was safe for the monarchy and probably wanted to remain that way. A federation of princes, instead, would not arouse the suspicions of monarchical Europe. It would respect the rights of the ruling princes, and at the most would have to face only the opposition of Austria. And by some it was even hoped that Austria itself might eventually decide to surrender its unruly Italian subjects and find compensatory expansion in the Balkans.

The apparent simplicity and facility of realization gave the federal scheme its peculiar appeal from its first appearance at the end of the eighteenth century down to almost the eve of the proclamation of the Kingdom of Italy in 1861. It was the thesis advanced by Botta (1789), Angeloni (1814), Vieusseux (1822), before Mazzini's Young Italy entered the field and later by the more widely-known writers, Gioberti in his *Primato morale e civile degli Italiani* (1843), Balbo in *Le speranze d'Italia* (1844), and D'Azeglio in *Proposta d'un programma per l'opinione nazionale italiana* (1847). It remained vigorous even after the disappointing experience of 1848. Louis Napoleon's intervention in Italian affairs was also based on the idea of a federation—in which, of course, the pro-Austrian rulers in power would be replaced by princes of his family. A considerable segment of the republican group was also for a federation. Their inspiration came from the Swiss historian Sismondi, who, Mazzini related in his *Memoirs*, "from the conditions of his Switzerland, had been nursed on federalism, and he preached it as the ideal political regime to the numerous Italian exiles, especially Lombards, who were around him and were inspired by him. There was no one among them who had even a suspicion that unity was possible and desirable" (77 : 37). And indeed, Carlo Cattaneo, Ferrari, and, for a time, Montanelli, could not conceive an Italian republic not federative.[13]

Mazzini opposed federalism with a passionate, obstinate, tireless persistence, to which the defeat of Louis Napoleon's scheme of Italian federation must be credited as much as to the skillful maneuvering of Cavour. To him a federation, far from being an ideal type of organization, was at best a makeshift arrangement to be resorted to when local conditions did not permit complete uniformity of institutions, as in Switzerland, where the various provinces were different in language, religion, social customs, or in America, where great distances separated the centers of population. But even in federations experience had eventually shown that a closer union was necessary for the functions of government; it had been so in ancient Greece, where, Mazzini wrote, "the Greek republics pushed so far the obligation of uniformity in laws that was incumbent on the federated states, that the independent nature of the federation was ultimately changed"; and it was so in America where a federal *union* was sought by means of a gradual rapprochment to unity of laws, institution, fundamental principles (*3* : 261).

That the federal system is a necessity—we will not say in the United States because the comparison made between a continent extending over 1,570,000 square miles, and a peninsula of 95,000 square miles, is exceedingly ridiculous—but in Switzerland where two religions and three different languages are butting one another, we can understand. But in Italy? In Italy where for over three hundred years all public life has been extinguished, where for over three hundred years all groan under an equal weight of servitude? In Italy where, after our masters have forcibly joined parts exactly where there was greater dissimilarity of tendencies, there are no longer any divisions except, as in some cities in Romagna, within the confines of the same city? There no longer exists today, we make bold to assert, any difference in character or customs between one part of Italy and another, which is not found equally strong in France, between the departments of the North and those of the South, or in the British monarchy, between England and Scotland. There is not a single local interest with which organic unity is conflicting; there is not a single city that contends the privilege of the central power to the prophetic majesty of Rome. The very few who are eager to prepare the ground for an aristocratic influence, more easily implanted in a restricted sphere, are in favor of the idea of a federation (*25* : 262–63).

The example of America was sometimes mentioned by the advocates of an Italian federation. Angeloni, in his *Italy at the End of 1818*, suggested exactly a federation patterned after the United States of America. Later, in the early fifties, the publicist Angelo Brofferio, criticizing one of the many unitarian manifestoes issued by Mazzini, pointed out again that the future Italian state had to make provisions for the local convictions, interests, pride of the various Italian provinces and concluded: "We also want unity, but ... the unity of the United States of America, not that of England oppressing Scotland and Ireland, not that of Russia crushing Poland" (*45* : xiv).

To Mazzini the comparison between Italy and the United States was ridiculous because of the differences in geographical, historical, social, and religious conditions between the countries. In his *Dell'Unità Italiana* (On Italian Unity), he analyzed these differences and concluded that although the federal system was acceptable for America it was neither necessary nor desirable for Italy.

Two dangers, he thought, are apt to beset a federation, one from without and the other from within its boundaries: attacks from foreign foes, encouraged by the loose bonds of the federation, and the establishment of an aristocracy, even an untitled one, which may seize the government of the local units and control the federation through them. These two dangers were minimized in the United States by fortunate historical and geographical circumstances. The country was reasonably safe from foreign attacks, because of the protection afforded by the Atlantic Ocean. The establishment of an aristocracy dangerous to the republican liberties was perhaps beginning in America, but would still need a long time to establish itself firmly.

The aristocracy of conquest is formed suddenly by the apportionment of the land. But, where it does not rise from this cause, it is formed slowly and gradually with the accumulation of wealth, transmitted from father to son, or with the transmission of land and local prestige within a given territory, which little by little are concentrated in the more powerful families. Two generations have passed since the Declaration of Independence, and two generations are not enough to set up an aristocracy in the midst of a people that is young, risen out of a long popular revolution, not wasted by corruption, safe from the craft of neighboring aristocracies and tyrannies (*3* : 289).

But the mood, temper, and habits of Europeans in general, and Italians in particular, were quite different.

We are decayed, grown old in the habit of servitude, surrounded by enemies powerful in hatred and craftiness, and if today we aspire—and we shall succeed—to rejuvenate ourselves, the habits of our old age will hover over us for a long time, ready to renew their hold on us, if an opportunity is left open to them. So are we, and so is all Europe: the aristocracy of wealth in France did not need two generations to replace that of blood (*3* : 289).

A further and more obvious contrast between Italy and America was afforded by the geographical differences: the United States spread over a great expanse of territory, at that time already well over one and one-half million square miles, while Italy had an area of less than 100,000 square miles; the former included in its territory large lakes and vast deserts which hindered rapid communication, while the latter was thickly populated almost uninterruptedly from one end to the other. The fact that a single

state had not been established in America over a territory two-
thirds the size of Europe was no valid argument against the establishment of one in Italy, which was only one twenty-ninth of
Europe. The United States, Mazzini felt, was large enough for
many independent states as large as Italy.

Finally, there were differences in historical development which
made the federal organization in America not the result of a free
and deliberate choice but of necessity. The twenty-four United
States had come into existence as colonies at different times, with
different charters, and had been settled by different types of immigrants.

They differed in religious belief. They differed in types of organizations.
They remained for a long time under the control of England in varying
degrees. Some received both Governor and Council from London,
others only the Governor; some others needed only to change their
names at the time of the Revolution—so great was the liberty they
enjoyed under the charter granted by the government. Rhode Island is
still governed by the charter granted by Charles II; Connecticut changed
its constitution only a few years ago, in 1818. For others still, the
Revolution was a question of internal and external liberty at the same
time. To the differences in climate, soil, and customs, are to be added
those in the origin of the population and the economy of the regions.
The population of the Northern States comes from England for the
most part; that of the Southern States from the native descendants of
the early colonists. The plantations of the South subsist on the work of
the slaves; religious opinions instead tend to emancipation in the North,
and forbid slavery in New England. All these influences continued to
exert their power even after the great work of independence had been
achieved in common—and it was necessary to yield to the rivalry of
the States and build a neutral city for the seat of Congress. They are
still operative, waiting only for an occasion to assert themselves. We
heard, not long ago in [South] Carolina the firm assertion of the principle that popular sovereignty confers on every federated state the right
to renounce to the benefits and duties of the association, and to withdraw, when its own interest requires it: a principle which is sufficient
to cast once, to have it germinate and reappear later. This principle
seems to us an irrefutable truth, and offers therefore the strongest
argument against the federative bond, if applied to countries that must
and wish to form a permanent union. (*3* : 291).

Of course some of the differences, it could have been pointed out,
existed as well among the various regions of Italy: the monarchi-

cal South differed in political traditions from Central Italy, and
even more from Venice and Genova—oligarchic republics till a
few decades before. They differed widely in cultural level and
economic development. But Mazzini, for his polemical task, preferred to ignore the differences, and to reassert the essential unity
of Italy.

But with us—let us repeat it once again—where are the differences we
have just been detailing? Travailed by the same vicissitudes, educated
during the golden centuries to common glories and common liberties,
then to common servitude, oppressed, no province excepted, by the
same tyranny, subject to similar needs, which of the causes which precluded unity to America prevent it to us? It is necessary to come down
on Italian ground, and renounce the fallacies of examples (*3* : 291–92).

But although Mazzini rejected the example of America for a
federal organization of Italy, there were numerous points on
which he considered American organization, political traditions,
and customs well worth imitating. America's example could be followed in the organization of the small units of local government,
the townships (*3* : 333–34), in the call of a constitutional conven-
tion at the very birth of the new country (*6* : 52), in the opposition
of public opinion to secret diplomacy (*6* : 397), and in the way of
waging revolutionary war by guerillas (*3* : 213). Later, as his
knowledge of things American increased, he pointed out the
"consecutive ability that has been called to the Presidency of the
United States" as proof of wise choice of executives made by a
free people (*17* : 269); he repeatedly pointed to America as an
example of republicanism and assigned to America the "mission"
of teaching republicanism to the world (*83* : 165–67); he sought
information on the American educational system, both on the elementary and university level (*71* : 244–45); and he quoted with
admiring approval an unnamed American who, when asked what
regulations were there in his country to govern the freedom of
association, replied that they might as well ask him what government regulations were there limiting the freedom of breathing
(*75* : 304). In one of his last writings he even granted America the
role of nation-guide, which he so vigorously and persistently
denied to France.[14]

America appeared in still another role in Mazzini's mind—as a
place of deportation of European patriots. After the revolutions

of the thirties, western and central Europe used America as a dumping ground for their political undesirables, as Russia was using Siberia. Polish and Italian refugees in Switzerland, France, and Belgium were herded together and shipped to America, where their plotting against their home governments would be totally futile. On his accession to the Austrian throne, Ferdinand I issued an imperial rescript granting a commutation of sentence to a certain category of Italian political prisoners held in the Spielberg on condition that they agreed to be deported to America. A number of them—Confalonieri, Foresti, Borsieri, Castiglia, Tinelli, and others—accepted the condition, while "others preferred to wait in prison for the expiration of the sentence" (*11* : 124). This system continued for the next two decades, and as late as the middle and late fifties—just before the unification of Italy—political prisoners from Lombardy, Tuscany, the Papal states, and the kingdom of Naples were deported to New York.[15]

These deportations moved Mazzini to intense indignation because of the arbitrary manner they were decreed and the remote place of destination. That the refugees were received with kind hospitality and sympathy in America, Mazzini did not know at the time (1836) and perhaps did not care. America, end of the line of the deportees' journey, did not evoke in his mind the vision of the land of the free, the country of Washington and Franklin, but rather of a place where the exiles were denied the only comfort still left to them in Switzerland, "to look at the Alps or the Rhine, and think that their country was lying just beyond" (*13* : 128). His indignation was most bitter against Switzerland because republicans there, with base servility to the neighboring tyrannies, agreed to be a party to that "organized trade of white slaves" against their foreign brethren whose only crime was love of their country and its freedom. The truth of the matter was that the patriots, however noble, were using the territory of the Swiss republic to plot revolts and even armed invasion of neighboring countries, causing annoyance to the neighbors and embarrassment to the Swiss. This was true of Mazzini himself, who in 1834, with a band of Polish and Italian republicans, invaded Savoy with the intention of starting a revolt there. The attempt failed, and a search was begun for the apprehension and expulsion of the Italian conspirator—a search that failed, in spite of the 500 francs reward offered, partly because of the half-hearted way the local authorities of the cantons conducted it, partly because of the life of virtual prisoner Mazzini led to avoid capture, "in order not to give his family the grief of hearing of his deportation to America" (*12* : 246).

It must have been this "America," concentration camp for patriots, that Mazzini had in mind when in a letter to a friend in 1838 he said: "Do me the favor not to speak of America: I feel a cordial antipathy for the very name of that country" (*15* : 57).

CHAPTER II

YOUNG ITALY IN AMERICA

By 1833, Young Italy, the new secret society founded and directed
by Mazzini, had spread all over Italy and was ready for its first
trial of strength. The first attempt was a conspiracy to seize the
Piedmontese government and force the King to declare war on
Austria; but in the Spring of 1833, before the rising could take
place, the plot was discovered and crushed without mercy. A few
months later, in February, 1834, Mazzini attempted the already
mentioned invasion of Savoy; but even that second attempt failed,
partly because of the ineptitude or treachery of General Ramorino,
the military leader of the expedition.

Undaunted by these failures Mazzini redoubled his efforts to
strengthen and broaden the organization of the party. He founded
Young Europe (1834) to spread the principles of Young Italy among
the other European oppressed nationalities, especially the German
and the Polish; he published the biweekly paper *La Jeune Suisse*
(1835–36) until it was suppressed by the Swiss government; and he
continued until 1836 the clandestine publication and distribution
of the pamphlets of Young Italy. Sought by the Swiss police,
beset by plots of French, Sardinian, and Austrian spies, he succeeded for over two years with the aid of numerous Swiss sympathizers in avoiding arrest and deportation by moving constantly
from canton to canton, from village to village, from house to
house, at times fleeing by the back door while the police was knock-
ing at the front door. At length, when that hunted life began to
tell on the health of his two companions, Giovanni and Agostino
Ruffini, he consented to leave Switzerland. Crossing France with a
safe-conduct, on January 12, 1837, he reached England, the country that was to become his second homeland, where he was to
spend most of his remaining years.

The early period of his residence in England was one of great hardship, both physical and spiritual, during which the organization of both Young Italy and Young Europe disintegrated for the want of his leadership. But after a while he became acclimatized to the English atmosphere, regained his spiritual balance, and between the end of 1839 and the beginning of 1840 he took up again his political work. The first task he undertook was the reorganization of Young Italy, and for that purpose he contacted his friends on the Continent.

The friends most active in this work of reorganization were Giuseppe Lamberti and Pietro Giannone in Paris, Federico Campanella in Marseilles, and Luigi Melegari in Lausanne, four young patriots about Mazzini's own age, all compromised because of their revolutionary activities in 1831. He kept the closest contacts and most active correspondence with Lamberti, who, as Secretary of Young Italy in Paris, compiled and preserved an accurate record of all the correspondence passing through his hands from 1841 to 1848—a record later published as *Protocollo della Giovine Italia* which gives some interesting details on the activities of Young Italy in America.

The reorganized Young Italy had substantially the same structure as when it was first founded in 1831. It differed, however, in two important respects: it planned to organize patriotic Italians all over the world, not just in Italy, and to make its appeal not only to the educated middle class, as it had originally, but also to the working class. The system of recruiting followed Mazzini's usual plan: the appointment of a committee for each country which in turn was to appoint dependent committees for the provinces and so down the line: "Organize abroad a central committee for each country," he advised, "one for France, one for Spain, one for Switzerland, one for the United States, etc.; organize it from above, that is, not on my orders, or any one else's, but, as it happens in all things of this kind, by prevailing on the men best in mind and character, to make themselves the animators and the movers" (*19* : 414).

His friends objected to the new features of the scheme. Campanella felt that "Young Italy abroad is a simulacrum of association to delude Italians at home" and that it was necessary "only to be concerned with the general design, that is, to prepare the cadre of the army, securing honest, intelligent leaders in every place,

without worrying about rank and file followers, who undoubtedly
would be available when needed."[1] Also, Lamberti objected to
Mazzini's project "to gather the Italians abroad in a single association, no matter where they are, even in America, even at the
Pole, if any Italians should be there" (*19* : 99). Campanella expressed the fear that Mazzini was changing the essentially revolutionary character of the association: "Pippo [Mazzini] is concerned with the *thought* and forgets the *action*," he wrote to Lamberti. "He seems to consider the Association as something purely
academic, and not as an association preparing for a movement.
He wants to give a renown to *Young Italy*, to make its name
resound in all parts of the globe, rather than to organize it for the
action, as he should. He writes seriously to me that Congregations
are established in North America, South America, Constantinople,
Africa, etc. . . . The important point is inside Italy: it is from
there that must come the liberty of Italy, not from the Mississippi"
(*20* : 99–100).

Mazzini defended his decision with the argument that only by
giving evidence of vitality abroad could they hope to revive the
association at home. In addition, any work of propaganda required
funds, and those funds could be obtained only by organizing the
Italians abroad.

It is not true [he wrote to Lamberti] that I consider the principal part
of the work of Young Italy to be in America or in the Moon. But,
besides the work incumbent on us to educate Italians everywhere, I
need activity abroad in order to act inside Italy: I need to spread the
idea we are strong; I need a noise here to get an echo there; I need a
press above all, and you have no press without money. You cannot get
money from Italy before you are strong, so you must raise some outside,
and you cannot raise it without contributions, and you cannot get
contributions without an association. From the Congregation of New
York, which makes Federico *laugh*, I received the other day eight dollars, the price of one hundred copies of the *Apostolato*, and I swear to
you that I am most grateful to the American Congregation, for having
done more than all European congregations, London excepted. On the
other hand all points, even the most distant, are *Italian* to me when, as
in the case of New York, they are frequented by so many sailors from
Genoa and Leghorn. I fear no one of you has understood, till now,
either myself or my thought, and what is the importance of the work
abroad. I am perfectly convinced, like Federico, that Italian liberty
must come from Italy and not from the Mississippi; but I wish he

would show me how to act *directly* on all the Italians in Italy, and how to convince them, by means of mere argumentation, that they must conspire (*20* : 98).

Mazzini had good reasons to insist on including the Americas in his plan of reorganization. Even when Young Italy was almost paralyzed by the debacle in Savoy, Italian patriots remained active in South America. In 1835, he had heard from "an Italian association, an offshoot of ours, made up of business men, etc., founded in America, with center in Rio de Janeiro, translating items from our journal, and asking regular correspondence with me" (*10* : 378). In April, 1836, the first issue of the journal *Giovine Italia* was published by the Italians in Rio. Garibaldi, who had arrived there a few months earlier with letters of recommendation from Mazzini, had been warmly received by Italians who were wealthy enough and patriotic enough to equip for him a revolutionary flotilla of three boats, the *Young Italy*, *Young Europe*, and *Mazzini*, with which he annoyed the navigation of the Sardinian merchant marine. Garibaldi had even requested Mazzini, as if he were the head of a belligerent power, to supply him with letters of marque and reprisal so that he might pursue his patriotic endeavor as a privateer and not as a pirate.[2]

In North America also, a number of Italian patriots had found refuge during the last few years either voluntarily or through deportation, and some of them had been members of Young Italy. To mention only those closely associated with Mazzini, there were the two grand old men of the revolution, Giuseppe Avezzana and Eleuterio Felice Foresti, and two younger men, Giovanni Albinola and Alessandro Bargnani. Avezzana, a former officer in the Piedmontese army, who had once been sentenced to death for his revolutionary activities, had fought with the rebels in Piedmont in 1821 and later with the Constitutionalists in Spain. After a few years in Mexico, where he founded the settlement which became Tampico, he settled in New York City and operated a candle factory. Eleuterio Felice Foresti, once a lawyer and justice of the peace near Rovigo, had been imprisoned in the fortress of Spielberg and had been deported from there to America in 1836. At the time of his close association with Mazzini he was a Professor of Italian at Columbia College. Both of the younger men were in their thirties. Albinola had been a business man, and Bargnani a lawyer. Both had been arrested for membership in Young Italy in 1833, imprisoned in the Spielberg, and later deported to America. Mazzini did not know that two of these men, Albinola and perhaps Foresti, had shown weakness at their trials and had made revelations highly compromising to other revolutionists. He supposed that all of them were made of sterner stuff, and he must have felt that to ignore them in the reorganization of Young Italy would be an unforgivable waste of revolutionary talents.

The Central congregation for the United States was organized on June 6, 1841, shortly after that of London, and was directed by Felice Foresti, president, Giovanni Albinola, secretary, Giuseppe Avezzana, and Alessandro Bargnani. Its jurisdiction included, besides the twenty-five United States, Canada, Cuba, the West Indies, Columbia, Equator and Venezuela. Some organizers were appointed for the task of setting up local chapters, or congregations, of the Association in various centers: Dr. Pietro Bachi, Professor of Italian at Harvard, in Boston, Luigi Roberti, Instructor in Italian at Yale, in New Haven, Giuseppe De Tivoli, in Philadelphia, Carlo Bassini, in Richmond, Cristoforo Salinas, in Charleston, Dr. Natilj, in New Orleans, Giovan Maria Bonaccina, in Montreal, and Simone Sardi, in Venezuela (20 : 104).

The congregation of North America began immediately to establish contacts with the European congregations. On June 15, one week after their official establishment, they wrote to Mazzini, enclosing letters also for Lamberti in Paris and Campanella in Marseilles, to advise them of their constitution, to request regular correspondence, and to offer their services.[3] In order to maintain their high morale, Mazzini requested Lamberti, the clearing house of all the work on the continent, to send him two or three copies of any article published on Young Italy so that he might forward them to America (23 : 244, 258–59).

It is impossible to say how many congregations were actually active in the United States and how many never went beyond the stage of the appointment of an organizer. Foresti informed Lamberti on December 10, 1843, that besides the four congregations already existing in New York, Boston, New Orleans, and perhaps Philadelphia two more had recently been organized in Cincinnati and Louisville, "poor, however, in means and number, but important because through them the voice of Young Italy can reach the most remote sections of the Federation."[4] The Louisville congregation, however, though small, seems to have been zealous and generous, because two months later Foresti, writing again to Lamberti about a fund raising drive, informed him that "he had one hundred dollars from the Congregations of Boston and Kentucky: the others had not replied." In that same letter Foresti also reported the organization in New York of an Italian company of the National Guard consisting of forty uniformed men drilling under command of Avezzana.[5] Thanks to Albinola, who traveled extensively on business and made propaganda for Young Italy and its journal on the side, the order for copies of the *Apostolato* rose from one hundred to two hundred and finally to five hundred. Payments for these orders were often delayed, to the great distress of Mazzini, who had to meet the printer's bill with an empty treasury (*24* : 106).

Mazzini repeatedly expressed his satisfaction with the zeal and enthusiasm of the North American congregation, offering it as an example to the rather sluggish Parisian group. "For these brothers in New York," he wrote to Lamberti, "we can only have high praise. They proceed with much formality; they sent me a lithographed copy of the minutes of their meetings, of the appointment of organizers, etc. I am not very fond of formalities; but among us, unfortunately, it often indicates that things are taken a little more seriously" (*20* : 262). And to Lamberti again he wrote sometime later: "The work in the United States proceeds surprisingly well. In Boston the members of Young Italy meet regularly, wearing the national cockade, etc. Three agents have been sent by the Central Congregation of New York to organize in New Orleans, where [there] are several thousands of Italians. Another travels through the Antilles. I am mentioning these facts as an indication of the activity shown by our brethren there" (*23* : 74). A few days later he wrote to Giambattista Cuneo, president of the congregation of Montevideo, urging him to establish contacts with the New York group and reach an understanding with them for the organization in South America.

The Central Congregation of New York directs the work of Young Italy in the United States in an exemplary manner. ... The work of that Congregation proceeds with an activity and regularity that leave nothing to be desired. ... The tone of their correspondence assures me that Young Italy will some day obtain great benefits from North America (*23* : 90).

One effect of the activity of the New York congregation was to call Young Italy to the sympathetic attention of American liberals. Foresti, in a previously mentioned letter, informed Lamberti that *"The Democratic Review* and the newspapers *Sun* and *Evening Post* are ours, if we need them."[6] Mazzini in his letter of October 22, 1841, announced jubilantly to his mother:

A monthly review of New York, America, entitled *The Democratic Review*, contains, in its September issue, a long article on the *Apostolato Popolare* and our association, full of praise and declarations of sympathy on the part of the American democracy. A Miss Sedgwick, an American writer, in a book of travels on the continent, has also spoken of the first issue of the *Apostolato*. It seems that from the Americas the sympathy will pass on to the old continent (*20* : 344–46).

The following week he gave the same information to Lamberti, concluding, "Be patient a while, and you will see that the sympathies will be extended from country to country" (*20* : 350). This was an exhortation that failed to dispel the pessimism of Lamberti, who replied: "Very well about the American sympathy, but who will hear about it in Italy? It seems to me, on the other hand, that the procedure is a bit too long."[7]

Mazzini was understandably delighted with the article in the *Democratic Review*[8] since it was indeed very sympathetic to his views and unusually well informed on the revolutionary trends in Italy during the preceding decade. The author praised the Society highly for its spirit, "which, without profanity, we may call kindred to that of the apostle of old," for its "liberal principles" and "pure morals"; its journal, *Apostolato Popolare*, was found "replete with a true political wisdom, with sound and healthy views, pervaded with a high tone of pure Christian morals." Young Italy was contrasted favorably with its predecessors for its faith in the common people, who had been neglected and distrusted by the Carbonari; its political creed was expounded faithfully and in detail, and with expressions of approval. On one point alone the writer expressed a reservation. This was on Mazzini's uncompromising opposition to the federal system, but the reservation was presented with modesty and deference.

... we would suggest to their most careful consideration the practical study of the federative principle, in its working in our great republican union of republics. We will not here criticize the arguments which they derive from past history and present conditions of the country for which they are so much better competent to judge than we can pretend to be. But, in passing, we may be allowed to express to them our own profound confidence, that the federative principle, wisely applied to the organization of a union of independent republics, with distinct collective and national sovereignties, and a proper and well defined distribution of their respective subjects of national and municipal powers and duties, accompanied with a strong sentiment of national patriotism and love of the Union, is the most wise, firm and energetic form of government ever yet attempted among men,—a form, too, which would seem to us peculiarly adapted to the historical, geographical and political circumstances of Italy. On this point, however, we repeat that we do not feel entitled to sit in judgment upon the counsels of such body as the Society of which we speak. We content ourselves, as free Americans, and brethren to the friends of freedom everywhere—still more, to its martyrs!—with the expression of a most earnest hope that the *Giovine Italia* may, before no very distant day, triumph over its enemies, and witness and perform the realization of all its high patriotic and philanthropic aspiration;—and that Italy, so fair and so lovely in its very chains, so great still even in its most abject abasement, may yet assume, within the epoch of our own day, its just and elevated place among the nations of the earth.[9]

Mazzini commented in print on the paper published by the *Democratic Review* in the article "Encouragements to the *Apostolato*," in which, after relating the popularity achieved by the journal among the Italians in North and South America, he discussed the American publication.

Not only the Italians but also the American republicans encourage our word. The *Democratic Review*, ... published in New York, in its issue of September, 1841, devoted a long article to the *Apostolato Popolare* and *Young Italy*. After an historical narration of the first period of the life of the association, and a faithful exposition of its political principles, the Review expresses the most unlimited approval—except on the principle of unity about which the writers propose some doubts, natural for those who live under a federal organization—and exhorts all Italians to rally under its flag. "With a cordial expression," we are translating the words of the Review, "of the sympathy of the American democracy, we can only wish to its worthy conductors that reward which is their own highest aim—the rapid extension of the number of their converts and brethren, and the speedy advent of the day which we are well assured is destined to witness the triumph of their high and holy cause, the emancipation of their beautiful country, its restoration to its natural position in the great family of nations, and its enjoyment of the blessings—inestimable amidst all their worst drawbacks—of freedom and democracy. May the mass of the Italians become but well embued with the truth of the doctrines to which the love of their patriotic brethren is thus striving to direct them, and assuredly the consummation of their mission, and the arrival of the fated hour, the wheels of whose car they are thus laboring to expedite, cannot be far."

About the doubts suggested concerning the unitarian system, we shall have occasion to talk, and we will show the American writers why the special conditions of the peninsula, and our past, compel us to unity. Today we only wish to thank them and assure them that their declaration of sympathy will give us strength to go forward in the midst of the obstacles that block our path, and that it affords us a new proof of the unity of the democratic faith, in which we are brethren.

May such expressions of sympathy be multiplied from country to country among the various fractions which make up the great democratic army! If each of us knew that he is working under the eyes of his brethren in faith—if, from nation to nation, the believers in Democracy shared efforts, praise, criticism—we would not see so many culpable discouragements, so many acts of bastard compromise, so much shameful impotence, as we still see today in our ranks (*20* : 345–46).

On the other American item Mazzini mentioned to his mother and friends—C. M. Sedgwick's *Letters from Abroad*—he was misinformed, because no reference is found in it to Young Italy or its publication, in spite of his categorical statement that "Miss Sedgwick quotes the first issue of the *Apostolato* in her *Letters from Abroad*" (*20* : 350). Catherine Maria Sedgwick visited England, Belgium, the Rhine Country, Switzerland, and Italy, in 1839 and 1840, spending most of the time in Italy. On her return she wrote her travel impressions in the *Letters from Abroad to Kindred at Home* to which Mazzini refers. The book was published in two volumes, the second of which is devoted entirely to Italy. In America she had known and befriended Confalonieri, Foresti, Gallenga, and other Italian exiles who gave her letters of introduction to prominent writers whom she later visited during her travels—Sismondi in Switzerland, Manzoni and Pellico in Italy. At Ferrara she visited with the family and friends of Foresti.[10] A woman of liberal ideas, she expressed in her book hostility to the tyrannical governments of the peninsula, sympathy for its people, and admiration for their culture. At the time of her journey Foresti had not established contacts with Mazzini; otherwise she would certainly have made his acquaintance during her stay in

London. Mazzini's erroneous statement can be explained with the hypothesis that he had not read her book but had only heard about it from his friends in America who perhaps wrote to him that it spoke favorably of the Italian patriotic movements, leading him to the conclusion that Young Italy must have been meant.

Another activity of the American congregations which gratified Mazzini was the institution in New York and Boston of schools for poor Italians patterned after the school he had himself founded in London a few months before. This school was started by Mazzini in 1841 for Italian children employed there as organ grinders by exploiters who recruited them in Italy with high promises and then held them in a state of quasi-slavery. Mazzini organized an association for their protection, and later founded a free school for them which was open evenings and Sundays. The school was supported by a number of his British friends, and it prospered until 1848, in spite of the opposition of Father Baldaccone, the chaplain of the Sardinian chapel in London. The inauguration of this school was announced in the *Apostolato Popolare*. Shortly afterwards a similar school was organized in Boston by Professor Bachi of Harvard, the organizer of the Young Italy in Boston.

Pietro Bachi, born in Sicily in 1787, had received a law degree from the University of Padua. In 1814, he took part in the Murat expedition to central Italy, and, after Murat's defeat, went to exile in England. He came to America in 1825. Shortly after he arrived in America he was appointed Professor of Italian, Spanish, and Portuguese at Harvard. He held that position until 1846. As soon as he heard of the London school, he organized one like it in Boston. Mazzini reported on the Boston school to Lamberti (*23* : 73), to his own mother (*23* : 82), and to Cuneo (*23* : 90). Later he announced it in the fifth issue of the *Apostolato* as follows:

We announced in the fourth issue of the *Apostolato* the establishment in London of a free elementary school for Italians deprived of means, at 5 Greville Street, Hatton Garden. We announce today with grateful joy that a school, similar to that of London both for intentions and class of people contemplated, has been opened in Boston (United States of America) by Professor Bachi, an Italian from Sicily. The teaching is free, and includes reading, writing, and history, and takes place three times a week (*23* : 90).

After Boston the example was followed by New York, though the New York school, perhaps because of its more elaborate program, took a few months longer to organize. A public meeting was held to discuss ways and means to open schools in New York and other cities of the Union, following which "even some American newspapers expressed their sympathy, especially the *Evening Post*" (*23* : 141). An American association supplied them, free of charge, with a place with facilities for two hundred pupils and contributed coal for the winter (*23* : 380–81). In the ninth issue of the *Apostolato*, Mazzini was able to announce the opening of the New York school.

From the New York papers and from our correspondents we learn what follows: the free Italian school in that city was opened on October 6, 1842, following the decisions made at a meeting on September 29th. The program includes reading, writing, arithmetic, history, geography, and English language: it takes place daily except Saturday and Sunday, from six to ten in the evening. Toward the end of the year a course of lectures on Italian history is planned for Sundays, to be delivered by a man whose name honors the Italian exiles and Italy [Foresti]. The principal teachers are Mr. Attinelli and Mr. Emanuele Sartorio, both Italians from Sicily. The treasurer of the school is Mr. Giuseppe Avezzana; the secretary, Mr. Giovanni Albinola; the director, Mr. Foresti. The room, supplied free of charge by Americans, is located at 10 Duane Street. The number of pupils was almost forty at the end of September, and was increasing every day (*24* : 25–26).

Mazzini hoped that the example of London, Boston, and New York would soon be followed by the Italian communities in Paris, Lyons, Algiers, Barcellona, Constantinople, and Montevideo where large numbers of Italian workers resided (*25* : 123). He repeatedly urged his correspondents to organize schools of that kind, which were "the bud of the people, Italy in miniature, and a promise for the future" (*25* : 160). All his exhortations were in vain. No new school was opened by Young Italy, and, after that first year, nothing more was heard about the New York and Boston schools, indicating that perhaps even those went out of existence.

The tie between the American and the European congregations was strengthened by the brief visit Foresti made to Europe in midsummer of 1843. Mazzini was eager to impress Foresti with the European work, and wrote to his friends in Paris to give him a suitable welcome. He informed Lamberti that Foresti was fond of formalities and advised receiving him with some ceremony.

He suggested that, if possible, they hold a special meeting of the congregation, take Foresti to the workers' union, after pre-arranging a good attendance, and see that he had as little contact as possible with Italians unfriendly to Young Italy. "When he comes back to London I will have some propositions for him concerning America, which are important to me, and I would like to find him in a favorable mood" (24 : 193).

Foresti did not stay long in Paris, perhaps no longer than two or three weeks. On his return to London, Mazzini was his constant companion, and referred to him quite often in his correspondence during September. What the propositions were that Mazzini had for him is not explained anywhere, but most likely they must have been connected with raising of funds for the association and possibly with plans to finance a Polish insurrection that was to take place simultaneously with the Italian revolution and put Austria between two fires. After Foresti returned to America, Mazzini wrote and asked Lamberti to write also "to urge him and all our other members to contribute more than they seem disposed to do to the fund for the action" (26 : 26).

That question of contributions was a sore point with the association. Toward the end of 1844, Mazzini began a drive to collect a National Italian Fund of 150,000 francs, a war chest to be held in readiness for the day of the revolution, for which Foresti was the agent in the United States. The initial drive did not yield very good results. There is a record of only one remittance for one hundred dollars (28 : 267), though an additional fund may have been held in New York. In 1847 when the Italian crisis was looming on the horizon, Mazzini renewed his plea to Foresti for intensification of his efforts, admitting that he was "most disappointed in them collectively taken" (Appendix, 3 : 339). Foresti replied by giving a rosy picture of contributions "promised" in case of revolution in Italy, but insisted that those contributions were to be employed exclusively for the mobilization of the Italian patriots in the United States. Mazzini pleaded for a concentration of all the funds in London; he pointed out that most of the exiles were in Europe, not in America, that they had numerous Italian officers in Spain to bring back to Italy, and that, finally, there was the question of the assistance to be given to the Polish exiles for "an operation which would strike the flank of the enemy, and which, by promoting the insurrection in Lombardy, might decide the question at one stroke. I know I spoke to you about this in London, and it is a project worked out in detail since then" (*33* : 80–81).

Later Mazzini wrote again to propose the use of those funds for the transportation of Italian exiles from South America. Garibaldi had proposed a project which was the embryonic idea of his famous expedition of the Thousand of 1860. He had a thousand men with him—an Italian battalion of six hundred men and a Basque battalion of four hundred men. The men were eager to follow him to Italy, but unfortunately he had at his disposal only a schooner which could transport no more than 150 men. If they could charter a boat in New York for five or six hundred men and give funds to charter a third small vessel the entire Garibaldi legion could be brought to Italy. Also, Mazzini wrote, they should try to purchase one hundred Colt carbines for them. "Study among yourselves," Mazzini urged, "if there is a way to aid in the realization of this project, and let me know. We are not dealing here with doubtful elements; it is a corps which, commanded by a man of the ability and renown of Garibaldi, would serve as the nucleus for the insurrection of Naples or Sicily, unless circumstances should call them elsewhere; it is an operation that could be decisive" (*33* : 104). But not even this proposition was accepted, and Garibaldi returned a few months later to Italy with only 144 men on the schooner *Esperanza*.

Another congregation whose activities were mentioned by Mazzini was the one in New Orleans. On January 18, 1847, Mazzini wrote to his mother as follows:

On November 5th in New Orleans the Italians commemorated there, with an imposing ceremony, the memory of the patriots of the Italian nationality. The city sympathized so much with the demonstration, that they treated us as representatives of a nation already in existence, as foreign governments are treated. A salute of one hundred guns was fired in the morning, and all the population of the city went to visit the building where the ceremony was held. A great catafalque was set up; I have the design of it, and I would send it to you if it were not too bulky. There were speeches, hymns, etc. All the papers of New Orleans talked about it (*32* : 19).

The ceremony must have indeed been very imposing, if we are to believe the reports of the local press. Five New Orleans dailies carried stories of this celebration.[11] The most extensive coverage was given by *Le Courrier de la Louisiane*, whose writers were perhaps closer to Young Italy since they had published the year before an article on the Italian society which Mazzini thought flattering enough to send to his mother (*28* : *258*).

According to the stories in *Le Courrier*, on November 4, at 5:30 P.M. a salvo of one hundred guns was fired on the Place d'Armes. On November 5, the day of the celebration, a gun was fired every half hour from sunrise to sunset "to inform the inhabitants of the city that this was a day of mourning and grief for the friends and compatriots of the unfortunate victims of European despotism."

The ceremony took place at seven o'clock in the evening in the Rotunda of the St. Louis Exchange, which had been especially decorated for the occasion. In the center of the Rotunda rose a catafalque on a base three feet high, on the four sides of which were inscribed four legends: "Ai Martiri della Libertà Italiana," "Exoriare aliquis nostris ex ossibus ultor," "Ora e Sempre—5 Novembre 1846," and "Et si religio jusserit signemus fidem sanguine." The upper gallery and the tribunes were decorated with back drops of black drapery surmounted by silver larmes. Against the sixteen columns which rose from the upper gallery to support the rotunda were placed sixteen shields, eight of them each bearing the name of one of the eight Italian states, the other eight, placed alternatively with the first, inscribed with mottoes of Young Italy—"Dovere," "Umanità," "Indipendenza," "Libertà," "Egualità," "Progresso," "Fraternità," "Unità."

The ceremony opened with the "Grand Overture" from Bellini's *Norma*. It was followed alternately by speeches and by other musical numbers: a "Largo appassionato" and a "Rondo" by Beethoven, a "Musical Chorus" by Mendelssohn, and finally a "Prayer" by Chopin. During the music the Italians paraded slowly around the monument. Speeches were delivered by Mr. Dimitry in English, Mr. Santini in Italian, and Messrs. Natilj and Marigny in French. U.S. Senator Pierre Soulé, who was to give an address in French, was unable to attend because of illness. "But if he was hindered," wrote the English reporter of *Le Courrier* in a quaintly gallicized English, "from making the sound of his eloquence be heard in the midst of his fellow-citizens and friends, so often listened with delight when advocating the cause of freedom and liberal principles—still, in the quiet of a sick chamber, we are persuaded, his aspirations were directed to the success of the holy cause of Italian Liberty." The rites were concluded with a grand funeral chorus for tenors and bassos especially composed for the occasion by maestro Gabici with words by Mr. Calcaterra.

The doors of the Exchange were thrown open at six, and in a short time the hall was filled to overflow. The *Daily Picayune* reported that the "galleries were thronged to excess and many hundreds of ladies and gentlemen were forced to leave, being unable to find room." The reporter of the *Daily Tropic* found "the Rotunda and the passageways leading to it so crowded that we could only look in." The reporter of the *Daily Delta* was not able "to gain even an entrance to the area that surrounds the monument or cenotaph. We have never before witnessed such a living mass congregated, or rather jammed, into one hall. The spacious bar room of the Exchange, outside, was also densely thronged with citizens unable to gain entrance into the Rotunda, and on all the principal streets leading from the Exchange might be seen hundreds, many of them ladies, returning at an early hour, and venting their regrets at being unable to witness the solemn and imposing spectacle." To accomodate visitors who had failed to gain admittance the evening of the celebration, the Rotunda remained open on the next two days and evenings. When Mazzini read the reports of the interest and enthusiasm of the people of New Orleans, he must have marveled at the inability of his friends to obtain financial contributions for the cause in that city.

One may wonder whether similar demonstrations were conducted by other congregations in America, the stories of which may be buried in the files of old newspapers. It is possible, of course, but not likely. If any had taken place, the news would have reached Mazzini, and he in turn would have promptly reported to his friends on the Continent these signs of activity of the association in far away America.

With the beginning of revolts in Italy early in 1848, Mazzini realized that the basis of Young Italy had to be broadened to appeal to patriots who might fail to share the intransigent republicanism of the society. On March 5, 1848, Young Italy was dissolved and was replaced by a "National Italian Association" which left all constitutional questions to be decided by the Italian people after they had achieved their freedom. Foresti was advised of this transformation of the party on March 17 and invited to direct its reorganization along the new lines (*35* : 42–43). In all likelihood this was not done, since most of the Italian patriots in America returned to Italy to take part in the struggle for independence.

Chapter III

THE CHRISTIAN ALLIANCE

UNTIL 1842, Mazzini's American connections were limited almost exclusively to Italian patriots residing in this country. He met few Americans up to that time or attached little significance to those meetings, because he either did not mention them at all or referred to them only casually in his correspondence. In a letter to his mother he related meeting at the Carlyles' Amos Bronson Alcott, whose theory of world regeneration through vegetarianism he found highly amusing (*23* : 230–31). In another letter he mentioned meeting a wealthy couple from Boston who expressed great admiration for the character of the Italian exiles they had known in the United States. Because the wife spoke Italian, he hoped to interest them in his school, the first anniversary of which was to be celebrated in a few days (*23* : 316).

Later in that year, however, through Young Italy in America Mazzini began to establish more interesting and important contacts with some American groups and associations sharing, for different reasons, his hostility toward the Papacy. The first indication is found in a letter informing Lamberti of preliminary accords made for an alliance between Young Italy and some Protestant associations in the United States which promised considerable moral and financial support for the work of Young Italy, especially in the Papal states. The efforts of Young Italy to organize a school for poor immigrants in New York must have come to the attention of Protestant leaders in that city who became interested in their effort and conceived the plan to organize similar schools in other localities all over the world where Italian exiles and immigrants might be located. The school in New York was opened, as previously mentioned, on October 6, 1842, in a building given free of charge by some Americans.

The early forties was just the time when great alarm was felt by many Protestants over the large influx of Catholic immigrants in the United States. The Native American associations opposed to the political activities of foreign born citizens in general and Catholics in particular were rising rapidly in many American cities with large foreign born population. The power of these groups reached its height with the election of a Native American as Mayor of New York in 1844. The fear was seriously entertained in some quarters that the Papacy was deliberately "infiltrating" America with a large immigration from Catholic countries in pursuance of a scheme for taking over the country politically and religiously. A petition to Congress from Washington County, New York, asked "whether this union of Church and State, this allegiance to the Pope, did not require legislation; whether there was not in operation, under the Leopold Foundation, a plan for the over-throw of our civil and religious liberties, and whether this was not to be effected by the emigration of Roman Catholics from Europe, and their admission to our right of suffrage."[1]

Although there is no evidence that Mazzini's Protestant American allies were connected with the Native American movement, there is no doubt that they were part of the emotional climate that fostered the growth of that movement.[2] To alarmed Protestants it must have seemed a heaven sent opportunity to use this association of Italians who were eager to fight the same enemy and able to carry the fight to the enemy in the Roman states themselves.

The ostensible purpose of the alliance was to diffuse instruction among the Italians by establishing free schools similar to those already organized in London, Boston, and New York by Young Italy in other cities of North and South America, Europe, and the Near East and by smuggling forbidden books into Italy from depots set up at convenient places along its borders. For the schools, the American society was to supply the funds, leaving the actual direction in the hands of Young Italy. For the operation of book smuggling, we may assume that Young Italy was to con-tribute the "know-how" and facilities they had developed through years of experience in smuggling patriotic literature across the frontiers of the Italian states.

But behind this avowed purpose there was a secret understand-ing, hinted at vaguely in the first letter, about help to be given to the Italian revolutionists. "The officers . . . will be elected among

those Protestants who have fully grasped the meaning of the connection between the two associations, and they, using the authority which shall be granted to them, will help substantially our
work. The Society, meanwhile, will work to create everywhere,
through the periodical press, a public opinion favorable to our
cause" (*23* : 270). From private letters as well as from public
announcements made in the following two years, it is evident that
the substantial help hoped for was money and weapons for the
revolution. In a letter to Lamberti deploring a premature and
futile revolt in Romagna, Mazzini expressed regret that the movement had not been postponed to give him time for a propaganda
campaign in England and "also for one in America which, through
the Society now public and established, looked promising" (*24* :
233). Concerning the same event, he wrote to Ricciardi: "Only
yesterday I heard from some Americans, toward whom my efforts
have been directed, that if the revolt in Romagna continues, they
will give financial support" (*24* : 349). An unnamed correspondent was assured that "we will get from American patriots in
contact with us arms and money, but after the action has begun"
(*Appendix*, *2* : 298). In a circular he proclaimed that the "Americas, where Young Italy is already so powerful, will give the
Italian revolution, through us, material means, such as arms and
money, if necessary for the war" (*25* : 283). And in his *Plan for an
Insurrection in Italy* (1844) he reiterated as follows:

Powerful aid will come to us from the United States of America, where
a vast Association under the name of Christian Alliance, has already
been publicly organized to promote the Italian development. We have
promises from influential men to that effect, on condition that an insurrection hold the field for a few months among us. In America and
England the Italian cause is considered important today, because of
the fears aroused by the attempts of the Roman Court (*25* : 299–300).

Mazzini was fully aware that an open alliance with Protestant
groups might compromise him in the eyes of many Italians. He
assured Lamberti that the sole purpose of the "secret alliance"
was to overthrow the temporal power of the Pope and win recognition of the right of Italy to unity, liberty, and independence.

You know me and my religious beliefs which abhor equally Catholicism and Protestantism. What I hope for Europe and Italy is broader
than either. There is, however, a common ground—something that we

both want to destroy. We want to overthrow what exists now, and allow the individual conscience to express its belief freely. Beyond that, absolute independence. In a free Italy everyone may propose what he considers the Truth (*23* : 269–70).

But even in this limited field of coöperation, he was careful not to appear personally, and he let his friends in Paris decide what use, if any, to make of the information he passed on to them.

The American Philo-Italian Society was formally organized in New York on December 12, 1842. The statute of organization, the names of founders—among them Prof. Samuel F. B. Morse of telegraph fame—and an article by Theodore Dwight, Jr. were published in the *New York Observer* of January 21, 1843.[3] Mazzini was kept informed of developments. He passed on to Lamberti the information that the Philo-Italian Society had been organized, that they were conducting a drive for members and funds, and that a gentleman from Boston had already contributed five hundred dollars (*24* : 153). Lamberti, as usual, poured some cold water on his enthusiasm by pointing out that the "American Society may be fine, but I should like results here not there."[4]

According to agreements, one member from each of the two societies was to leave immediately on a tour to set up auxiliary state and county societies, and two more representatives were to leave later for Europe to initiate the work. The representative of Young Italy was Albinola, who, according to a letter from Foresti, was traveling at that time on personal business through the Southwest where he was "spreading the *Apostolato*, and [being] well received everywhere."[5] It is likely that in his travels Albinola took care of both his personal business and the joint affairs of the Philo-Italian Society and Young Italy. The organization of congregations in Louisville, Cincinnati, and New Orleans—places, one may recall, where strong Native American societies were active—may have been due to this joint activity.

There is something paradoxical about this friendly interest for a foreign group in a movement like the Native Americans which was tinged, to say the least, with xenophobia. But this fact will appear less strange if we recall that the "nativists" did not object to foreigners residing in the country, though they did object to their taking an active part in politics. The members of Young Italy were reassuring on that score, because their membership in a foreign revolutionary society proved that they were too engrossed in foreign politics and in ways and means of subverting it to have any political interest left for America. They were grateful temporary guests of the country. In addition, they shared the hostility to Catholicism as a political group. The enemies of our enemies need not be our friends to make convenient allies. Mazzini's broad humanitarianism would have been shocked by the narrowness of nativism, but it is doubtful that he had any knowledge of its essence; at any rate no indication whatever appears in his writings.

On May 12, 1843, a few months after its foundation, the Philo-Italian Society was transformed into the Christian Alliance. The new society remained, like its predecessor, predominantly a New York organization: its constitution prescribed that eighteen of the twenty-four members of the directing Board of Councilors were to be residents of New York or its vicinity. In 1845, only five councilors were from outside New York—three from Boston, one from Hartford, Connecticut, and one from Pennsylvania. A somewhat similar ratio prevailed also among the vice-presidents of the association—mostly presidents of affiliated societies of the Alliance—who were *ex-officio* members of the Board of Councilors. Out of a total of thirty, twenty-one were from New York City or State, and of the other nine, four were from Connecticut, two from New Jersey, one from Massachusetts and one each were from the more remote Louisville and Detroit.[6]

According to its constitution, the object of the Society was "to promote religious freedom, and to diffuse useful and religious knowledge among the natives of Italy and other papal countries." In order to explain why this object was important to all Christiandom and to state what means were contemplated for its attainment, the Alliance issued an address to all Protestants in America.

The Papal empire over the mind of man, the address stated, was still very extensive and closely allied with despotic governments. An intellectual and moral revolution that won for the Italians freedom of religion would weaken the power of the Papal system and would have beneficial results for all Christianity. After trying for the last twenty-five years to improve the political conditions of their country by means of violent revolutions, many Italians had come to realize that no change was possible in Italy until new ideas were diffused among the masses, until, the address stated, the "gay, unthinking peasantry of her villages, and the mechanics and shopkeepers of her towns begin to become inquiring thoughtful men." But, the address continued, "many of them having been made acquainted, by years of exile, with what it is that constitutes the happiness of nations truly free, have become convinced that the great charter of such happiness is the Bible, and that the ideas which are to work out the true emancipation of their country, can never be awakened in the masses, but in connection with the teaching of that book."

This situation gave the Alliance the opportunity to serve the cause of religious freedom throughout the world by helping the Italians. In spite of strict police measures, it was possible to introduce books in the Italian states. Many Italians living outside their country could be reached, and they in turn could reach their fellow-countrymen in Italy. Books in other languages could be translated by educated Italian exiles and later distributed throughout Italy. On these possibilities was grounded the specific program for which the Alliance solicited contributions. The Alliance proposed (1) to send "a judicious agent" to Europe, North Africa, the Near East, and, if possible, to Central and South America, to establish in localities where large numbers of Italians resided "a correspondence, and depositories for the sale of Bibles and other books, and to effect other arrangements for the religious and intellectual improvement of that interesting people"; (2) to prepare and publish Italian books and tracts, and to translate into Italian D'Aubigné's *History of the Reformation* and McCrie's *Memorials of the Reformation in Italy*; and (3) to prepare and issue a series of publications exposing to the American public the true character of the Papacy as a system.

With questions properly political [the Address concluded] our association has nothing to do. We do not undertake to persuade the people of Italy that their government needs reformation; that a republic is happier than a monarchy; or that an elective magistracy is better than a hereditary aristocracy. Whatever may be our judgment as individuals, whatever our sympathies as American citizens, we are not political propagandists. We only assert the sacred right, the religious duty of every man to read the Scriptures for himself, and to worship God, not in blind submission to priests or potentates, but in the exercise of his own faculties, and according to his own convictions.[7]

When Mazzini received the pamphlet containing the constitution and address of the Christian Alliance, he was disappointed. The

emphatic disclaimer of any political interest, the implied condemnation of revolutionary movements, the silence maintained over
the establishment of schools, except for the vague phrase, "other
arrangements for the religious and intellectual improvement of
that interesting people," were quite at variance with what he expected. When he sent the pamphlet to Lamberti, he mentioned the
idea of writing "an address in English to the Society, to correct
the errors which are found in their manifesto" (24 : 239), and he
repeated this intention in the notice of the foundation of the
Christian Alliance he inserted in the *Apostolato*.

We shall give in the next issue of the *Apostolato* some quotations from
an Address by the officers of Young Italy to the American Society.
We wished, in the meantime, to call the attention of our readers to this
new proof of sympathy, which comes to the Italian cause from a republican people who is powerful even today, and is destined to become
even more powerful with the abandonment of that policy of isolation,
suggested by necessity of circumstances to their first lawgivers. Some
of the opinions expressed in the Address betray an imperfect knowledge of our condition: it is up to us to rectify, and we shall attempt to
do so. But what is important is the affection with which the men who
dictated it look upon us, and the conviction that the free development
of the Italian element is necessary to the orderly progress of Humanity
(23 : 269–70).

The *Apostolato* ceased publication with that very issue, and the
address referred to was never issued. Mazzini, however, took
occasion to specify his objections to some of the ideas of the
Christian Alliance in a review of the pamphlet he wrote in 1845 for
The Westminster Review in which he stated that the plan of the
Association was good but incomplete, because it was solely
theological and because it failed to recognize frankly the political
requirements of the situation. It was true, Mazzini granted, that
the religious question was the most important. But how could a
people solve it unless and until they achieved political freedom?

Now, we acknowledge that in Italy, as everywhere else, the religious
question surpasses in importance all others; but we believe that sooner
or later the thinking world will be convinced that, in the present state
of the peninsula, it is impossible to get at the religious question otherwise than through the political. *To be* must precede *to think*; and Italy is
not. To aim at her present progress toward religious liberty would be
to impose the task of physical motion on a prisoner bound hand and

foot. You may warehouse Bibles, or copies of Merle D'Aubigné and McCrie at every point around Italy that may favor their dispersion; slowly and in numbers imperceptible, they may reach the hands of those who have no need of them, of those whose souls are already freed; but the mass, "the gay unthinking peasantry of the villages of Italy," "the mechanics and shopkeepers of her towns," will never hear of them. The gendarmes, the priests, and the Custom House form, between them and the instruction you seek to afford, a triple wall insurmountable to individual agents of a Transatlantic Society. Every theory of education, then, for the masses of Italy, resolves itself into a problem of liberty. And well do the patriots know this. Since the founders of the Christian Alliance wrote in their address that, "The patriotic minds of that glorious land are understood to have abandoned hope of liberating their country by insurrection and the sword," projects and attempts of that very order have multiplied in a frightful ratio(*31* : 86–87).

Though the Christian Alliance was too conservative to satisfy Mazzini, it was radical enough to alarm the Papal Court and to call upon it a pontifical condemnation. On May 8, 1844, Pope Gregory XVI issued an encyclical letter to "reprobate by name and condemn the aforesaid new society of the Christian Alliance constituted last year at New York, and other associations of the same sort, if any have joined it, or shall hereafter join it," and calling on the Patriarchs, Primates, Archibishops, and Bishops "to seize out of the hands of the faithful, not only Bibles translated in the vulgar tongue, published contrary to the . . . directions of the Roman Pontiffs, but also proscribed or injurious books of every sort" and exhorting to special vigilance the prelates governing churches "on the confines of Italy, or wherever emporiums and ports exist from whence there is frequent communication with Italy. For as the sectaries themselves propose to carry their plans into effect in those places, those bishops are especially bound to coöperate with us so as by active and constant exertion, with Divine help, to defeat their machinations."

In spite of the emphatic disclaimer of political intent by the Christian Alliance, the political implications of a propaganda for liberty of interpretation of the Scriptures were called by the encyclical to the attention of the rulers of the Italian states.

Such endeavors on your and our own part [continues the admonition to the Bishops] we doubt not will be aided by the help of the civil powers, and especially by that of the most potent princes of Italy; as well on account of their distinguished zeal for preserving the Catholic religion, as because it cannot have escaped their wisdom, that it is highly to the interest of the common weal, that the aforesaid designs of the sectaries should fail. For it is evident, and proven by the continued experience of the past ages, that there is no readier way to draw nations from their fidelity and obedience to their princes, than that indifference in the matter of religion, which the sectaries propagate under the name of religious liberty. Nor is this concealed by the new society of the "Christian Alliance"; who, though they profess themselves averse to exciting civil contentions, yet confess that from the right of interpreting the Scriptures, claimed by them for every person of the lowest class, and from the universal liberty of conscience, as they term it, which they would thus spread among the Italian race, the political liberty of Italy will also spontaneously follow.[8]

On May 12, 1845, when the Christian Alliance held its third annual meeting in New York the members were understandably elated over the attention the society had received in the Papal encyclical. It was the best possible advertisement they could desire, and they made use of it by publishing it together with the proceedings for that year. To them it was a proof that their plan of action had great possibilities of success, since the Catholic church seemed alarmed by the prospect. One of the speakers at the meeting, the Rev. Edward N. Kirck remarked: "Many here think the Alliance is a feeble affair. Well, sure, if anybody ought to know, it is His Holiness. The Priests of Rome do not conceal their costernation."[9]

In spite of reiterated disclaimers of political ends, the Christian Alliance was attacked by Catholic writers both in America and Italy for their unconfessed political aims. Their connections with Italian revolutionists—which must have been an open secret— were emphasized, perhaps to alarm contributors and supporters of conservative leanings. The *Freeman's Journal*, in an article entitled "Young Italy and her American Allies," asserted that, in contrast with the various bible and tract societies already in existence which "confine their operations to attempts at sectarian proselytism in an innocent and most harmless way, making decidedly more noise than work," the Christian Alliance was indeed "a politico-religious association. . . . Its political character, and the manifestation of such character it has already made . . . we deem obnoxious to the severest censure, as subversive of law, order, and that respect and deference which as *Americans* we *owe* to the municipal and police regulations of *neutral* states at amity and upon terms of reciprocal friendship with the United States." Passing under silence the principal avowed aim of the society, religious liberty, the writer analyzed the address to bring out the point that the purpose of the society was actually the same as that of the political revolutionist. It was, he pointed out, a moral and intellectual revolution which in turn would eventually bring about a social and political revolution. The means employed were different, to be sure, but since attempts at political revolution through violent means had failed, Italian revolutionists themselves agreed that the means contemplated by the Christian Alliance were appropriate to achieve *their own* aim. And the coöperation of "those expatriate specimen of Italian patriotism," was accepted and even sought by the Christian Alliance without inquiring into their religious views or inquiring whether they had any religion at all. "In other words," the article concluded, "the Christian Alliance has declared its *approval* of the scheme of Italian revolutionists and incendiaries; has established itself the associate and patron of political secret societies of Italian refugees; in fine, has become the friend and ally of 'Young Italy.' We presume, in charity, that the respectable portion of the members of the Alliance are unacquainted with the very peculiar character of this 'Young Italy,' and of the pranks which she has been playing during the last few years."[10]

Italian Catholics reacted in a somewhat similar manner. Father Giovanni Perrone, S.J., in his *Protestantism and the Rule of Reason* also attacked the Alliance for the political slant given to its propaganda. He did not fear Protestantism as a religious system, according to his American reviewer, because it was too cold for the Italian temperament. But he feared it as "a powerful instrument" in the hands of the Christian Alliance and the Italian "demagogues" "in the mad attempt at the establishment of democracy in Italy." Protestantism was presented by them to the Italians as *the* way to achieve political, civil, and social progress. The prosperity of Protestant America and England was pointed out as example of the benefits accruing from religious liberty. Father Perrone's thesis was that a good deal of the prosperity of those countries was only an appearance and that what was real was due not to Protestantism but to their Catholic heritage; hence a conversion to Protestantism for the sake of material progress would have been futile. Protestantism, "while it furnishes no means to attain eternal life . . . most miserably fails to fulfill its promises of political and civil amelioration in society."[11]

Curiously enough, on the basis of concrete achievements the Christian Alliance did not seem to deserve, at least in the first years of its existence, all the attention it received. The writer in *Freeman's Journal* assured his readers the Alliance had failed in its attempt to raise funds; that at the great rally held in 1844 at the Broadway Tabernacle, "notwithstanding the coaxing, wheedling, almost driving tones of Mr. Ketchum and a host of ministerial assistants, and, although a hat was actually passed around, not a cent could be raised to convert Italy."[12] That there was at least a measure of truth in this assertion was borne out by the report of the corresponding secretary of the Alliance at the 1845 annual meeting in which he admits: "It is not our privilege to report, as yet, very extensive results for the simple reason that we have been so far rather in a forming state. . . . As yet our organization has not been sufficiently known to secure the resources we need for the execution of our plans. The translation of Merle D'Aubigné's *History of the Reformation in Europe* has been commenced, and as soon as the requisite funds shall have been obtained, it will be completed, and the whole work printed. Our ulterior plans will be carried into execution as far and as fast as the circumstances will permit."[13]

Perhaps on account of these attacks by the Catholics, circumstances took a favorable turn for the Alliance, because later in that year they were able to send two of their agents—John McMullen and Alessandro L. Bargnani—to Europe to initiate their work. On September 9, 1845, they were in London and expected to be in Paris shortly. They remained in England, however, for several weeks, until the end of October, establishing contacts with local Bible Societies. During their stay in London they must have had frequent conferences with Mazzini, in the course of which the divergence in aim and method between the two associations must have become painfully clear—painful especially to Mazzini, who saw that Bargnani, a man who had suffered imprisonment at the Spielberg and life banishment in America because of his membership in Young Italy, had gone over completely to the Christian Alliance. A skeptical, ironic note seems to crop out in his letters from then on when referring to "Bargnani & Co." He announced their arrival to Lamberti as "those sent from America to biblicize and protestantize or reform Italy" (*28* : 129–30); he wrote to Raffaele Ciocci, a fellow exile in Liverpool: "Perhaps you have seen Bargnani, and have offered orisons in council that the Man of Sin be engulfed in the abyss" (*Appendix 3* : 55). He requested Lamberti to receive cordially Bargnani "an excellent person, with the fixed idea, as agent of the Christian Alliance, to wage war on the Pope with bibles and I don't know what else" (*28* : 176–77), but urged him and his other associates in Paris to speak to him always as members of Young Italy, to feel sympathetic with the aim of the Alliance but not share it, to be willing to supply useful indications, references, introductions but not take any active part in their work which "must proceed parallel to ours, without confusion and open league, with mutual sympathy and in agreement as to what we both must fight" (*28* : 182–83).

Bargnani made a better impression in Paris. Lamberti wrote favorably about him to both Mazzini and Foresti, and after his departure from France remained in correspondence with him, together with Giannone, for the next two years.[14] After two weeks in Paris Bargnani went to Switzerland and settled in Lugano, where he remained until the revolution of 1848 in charge of the book smuggling operation. McMullen visited Italy in the Spring of 1846. Bargnani wished to visit the Austrian provinces in Northern Italy, and had the American Ambassador in Switzerland request permission of Vienna, but permission was denied. While in Paris Bargnani prepared the prospectus of a newspaper, copy of which was sent to Giambattista Cuneo in Montevideo for circulation among the Italians there, which may have been the Italian weekly started in Paris at that time to advocate religious liberty.[15] Another newspaper, the *Maltese Indicator*, was started in Malta, perhaps also under the auspices of the Christian Alliance, by what the *Brownson's Quarterly Review* called "a wretched band of apostate friars and priests."

All these activities must have had considerable nuisance value, even though the number of converts made was quite small. The above mentioned Father Perrone admitted that "the faction calling itself the party of Progress, that is to say, the demagogy, waxed stronger and stronger; it dominated over Italy, and felt itself powerful enough to be insolent in Rome, the center and seat of Christianity. Tracts, cunningly prepared as arguments against

Catholicity and in favor of Protestantism, were distributed in great numbers by unseen hands. The Holy Father warned his people against the new plot designed for their ruin, and the Bishops of Italy, especially the Bishops of Tuscany, raised their voices to sound the alarm to their flock. But the warnings evoked by pastoral zeal were, for the moment, in too many places rendered inefficacious by the artifices of the demagogues."[16]

During the brief period of Mazzini's political ascendency as one of the Triumvirs of the Roman republic (1849), his friends of the Alliance flocked to Rome. Ferdinand De Lesseps, special French envoy in Rome, reported to his government that for several days he had seen Mazzini closeted with American and English missionaries, agents of political and religious propaganda (40 : 257–58). But this final contact was again mutually disappointing. The Alliance was undoubtedly disappointed by the deferential attitude Mazzini took in respect to Catholicism as the sincere belief of practically the whole Roman population; Mazzini was disappointed in the Protestant association for its failure to come to the aid of the Roman republic, whose constitution, while recognizing the *fact* that Catholicism was the religion of almost the totality of the population of the republic, also asserted the *principle* of freedom of worship.

Afterwards the contacts with Bargnani became tenuous to the vanishing point. There is no trace of correspondence with him until late in 1849, when Mazzini once again tried in vain to obtain some funds from the Alliance (40 : 289). Bargnani, on the other hand, by that time was definitely alienated from Mazzini. The year before he had published in Cattaneo's *Archivio Triennale* two articles advocating measures strenuously opposed by the republican leader: the immediate annexation of Lombardy to Piedmont, which to Mazzini's mind was the cause of the collapse of the revolution of 1848, and the coöperation of parish priests in a fight against the doctrines of "socialists, communists, and other sects equally delirious and irreligious,"[17] in which he most likely included the Mazzinists. And Mazzini later sadly commented to Foresti that Bargnani, Albinola, and the other members of the New York congregation who returned to Italy had all renounced their republican faith and accepted the principle of the regeneration of Italy under the leadership of the princes (42 : 14–15).

A last contact between Mazzini and American Protestants took place when Col. Hugh Forbes visited America. This Englishman had participated in the Italian revolution in Palermo, Venice, and finally in Rome, where he had been closely associated with Mazzini and Garibaldi. Early in 1850, he came to America "with the indefinite mission," Mazzini wrote to Foresti, "to evangelize the Americans in the sense of our ideas and hopes" (42 : 95). In February, 1851, he gave a series of public lectures in New York which was advertised and favorably reported in the press[18] and which was repeated by invitation at New York University the following month and later published in pamphlet form.[19]

In 1849, the Christian Alliance had merged with the Foreign Evangelical Society and the American Protestant Society to form the American and Foreign Christian Union.[20] Forbes approached this Protestant group, and, according to Foresti, since he was "very active, foresighted, a good speaker, skilful and convincing with his bland and courteous ways, and above all patient and persistent, he succeeded in impressing very favorably the Protestant ministers" who promised again to help the Italian revolution when the time came (42 : 65–66).

But in spite of Foresti's optimistic report, Forbes found that Protestant ministers were reluctant to acknowledge openly any interest in the cause of the Italian revolution. On May 12, 1850, the executive committee of the Christian Union issued an address to its members urging them to take advantage of the antipapal resentment in Italy over the French occupation of Rome for Protestant propaganda lest "Italy . . . be rescued from the grasp of Popery, only to fall into the jaws of infidelity." A number of young laymen in Boston, on Forbes' instigation, formed a society to further this work. They cautiously stated that although they sympathized with the political hopes of the Italian patriots their society "does not contemplate any direct action in the matter, but intends to limit itself to a *simple propagandist operation*."[21] But in spite of this caution, the preachers' meeting declined to endorse the society and passed a resolution stating that "while we would express no opinion unfavorable to the case in which Col. Forbes is engaged, nor interfere with the right of any member of this Meeting to coöperate with him, yet, as a Meeting, we think best to recommend no specific mode of action." And Forbes, astonished and chagrined, asked in one of his lectures: "Is the zeal of the Pilgrims sunk into apathy—or is the aversion to Popery, which formerly existed among the Puritans, now turned to sympathy? Will those who formerly protested against Popery, now protest against the revolutionists who strive to overthrow their enemy?"[22]

Mazzini does not seem to have had any further connection with Protestant groups, although he maintained friendly relations for a long time with some militant laymen such as Judge Thomas Russell of Boston and Col. Rush C. Hawkins of New York. The pact of cobelligerency between him and the American antipapal associations ended, as it was bound to end, in failure. Mazzini's immediate goal was political not religious reform. The religious reform he presaged for a distant future went far beyond the ideal of the sixteenth century reformers and envisioned a church truly catholic that would unite all believers, equate all faiths, and avoid with equal care the two extremes of Protestant "anarchy" and Catholic "tyranny."

Protestant clergymen on their part were understandably chary of close connections with Italian republicans. Churches are normally supported by conservative people who would naturally look askance at a league of the cloth with "red republicanism," the label which, rightly or wrongly, was pinned on Mazzini. Forbes shrewdly observed that the Italian problem was like a magnet with two poles, "the one being political attraction, the other dogmatic repulsion," and that "with some of the antipapal clergy, the political attraction was stronger than the repulsion upon dogmatic principles." The Albertine constitution in Piedmont, which allowed freedom of worship and free circulation of bibles and religious tracts, rescued the preachers from the uncomfortable dilemma. The Christian Union gave some financial aid and delegated the task of propaganda in Italy to the Valdensian church in Piedmont, feeling grateful to the House of Savoy that opened "a great door of usefulness . . . in the Kingdom of Sardinia,"[23] and wasting no more sympathy on the republicans.

But although devoid of practical results, the connection with the Christian Alliance was not without value to Mazzini. It certainly must have created an awareness, if not popularity, of Mazzini and his ideas in middle class America in general and militant Protestant circles in particular, a fact that perhaps a search through the files of the periodical literature and daily press of the middle and late forties could verify. At that time we begin to notice in Mazzini's correspondence frequent references to "American visitors," most of whom, unfortunately, are not more clearly identified. Among Americans who became acquainted with Mazzini and his circle at that time we find John L. O'Sullivan, editor of the *New York Morning News*,[24] and a Mr. Hawkes, "an American who sympathizes greatly with our cause, and who may help us a great deal" (*30* : 105), whose name recurs frequently in Mazzini's correspondence of 1846. American acquaintances at that time became numerous enough and trustworthy enough to be employed, together with Englishmen, as couriers or intermediaries for the clandestine correspondence Mazzini and his friends were maintaining with Italy (*30* : 245).

Of the American acquaintances Mazzini made at this time, the most important both for the eminence of the person and for the close friendship that later developed was Margaret Fuller.

CHAPTER IV

MARGARET FULLER

THE FRIENDSHIP of Mazzini was one of the most important influences in Margaret Fuller's mature life. It was the final turning point in her career as a writer and a crusader, a fact that has been duly brought out by all her biographers. "Here was a hero," says one, "who loomed as large to her as any of her beloved ancient Romans. She found him heroic, courageous, faithful, and wise. ... Under his influence her interest in the cause of the Italian exiles budded and then blossomed. It was the last and the greatest cause of her life, and she was to sacrifice everything to it."[1] "He was to her," writes another, "the new incarnation of the republican tradition which had been worshipped . . . in the Groton farmhouse. The defender of Brutus . . . had naturally developed into the disciple of Mazzini. The ideals that blazed forth in the fiery pamphlets of Young Italy she had long learned to reverence in Cambridgeport, when Timothy Fuller fared forth to air them in Fourth of July orations."[2] The references to Miss Fuller found in Mazzini's works do not alter or add much to this picture. However, they give details about their personal relationship which, though of minor importance, are not devoid of interest.

Even before they met personally in London in the Fall of 1846, they were not unknown to each other. Mazzini had heard of Miss Fuller from the Carlyles (*Appendix, 6 : 506*). Jane Carlyle was an admirer of the American writer whose *Woman in the Nineteenth Century* had recently been reprinted in England. Mazzini perhaps had heard of Miss Fuller also from Harriet Martineau, the English novelist who eleven years before had introduced Miss Fuller to Emerson[3] and who had been one of the first patronesses of Mazzini's free school for poor Italians.[4] Miss Fuller was undoubtedly acquainted with the name of Mazzini. She had reviewed for the

Tribune (January 6, 1846) the Boston *Liberty Bell for 1846*, an
annual to which Mazzini had contributed the antislavery item,
"A Prayer to God for the Planters, by an Exile." The activities of
the Christian Alliance and, even more, the scandal of the violation
of Mazzini's correspondence by the English postal authorities
with the lengthy parliamentary investigation and violent press
polemics resulting from the incident, had revealed Mazzini to the
American public as one of the most redoubtable champions of the
revolutionary cause. Thus, in her first correspondence from
Europe to the *Tribune*, Miss Fuller could refer to Mazzini as a man
well known to American liberals, "to those among us who take
an interest in the cause of human freedom, who, not content with
the peace and ease bought for themselves by the devotion and
sacrifices of their fathers, look with anxious interest on the suffering nations who are preparing for a similar struggle."[5]

In addition, Miss Fuller was acquainted with at least two persons who were in touch with Mazzini at that time—Pietro Bachi,
Professor of Italian at Harvard and organizer of Young Italy in
Boston, and the Dane, Paul Harro Harring, a curious type of poet,
idealist, adventurer, whom she met and befriended in New York.
Harring had participated in Mazzini's abortive invasion of Savoy
in 1834, and had been the historian of that adventure.[6] When he
later came to America, he made arrangements for the publication
of a novel, *Dolores*, in which Mazzini appeared as one of the characters. His publishers at the last moment refused to honor the
contract, and he appealed to Miss Fuller, at that time literary
critic of the *Tribune*, who lent him money to publish the story and
discussed his case in her column, suggesting the formation of
"congress of authors and publishers so that contracts would not
again be broken."[7]

Mazzini and Miss Fuller had in common numerous ideas, mostly
drawn from the French utopian socialists under whose influence
Mazzini had been in his early years in France and who had found
in America in the late forties an expounder and defender in Horace
Greely, Miss Fuller's friend and employer. Their thoughts on
religion, social justice, the role of woman in society were re-
markably similar. What they differed in was temperament.
Margaret Fuller at that time was still the cold, cerebral type, an
intelligence that gave light without warmth, while Mazzini was
of an ardent, emotional nature with ideas rooted in deeply felt

sentiments. Because of this contrast, Miss Fuller at first approached Mazzini with a critical reserve, as if she wished to study him, but her reticence soon gave way to almost complete surrender. "I remember poor Margaret Fuller," Mazzini reminisced many years later, "who came from the United States with I don't know what diffidence toward us. Led in our midst to one of those gatherings, after one hour she became our sister. Her soul, candid and open to all noble feelings, had divined the treasure of love which the religion of the Ideal had uncovered among us" (77 : 272).

Miss Fuller arrived in London at the end of September, 1846, together with Marcus and Rebecca Spring, well-known philanthropists and business associates of Horace Greely. When almost one-half of their six-weeks' visit to London had elapsed and no opportunity to meet Mazzini had occurred, she wrote him a note to which he replied (October 19) expressing regret for having been compelled "so long to postpone the pleasure of *her* personal acquaintance" and promising to call on her on the following Saturday, together with Harring (*Appendix*, 6 : 506–7). They must have met in the quarters she shared with the Springs in Golden Square, since his next note closed with "kindest regards to Mr. and Mrs. Spring." In the course of the evening Harring delivered himself of some unflattering opinions about the United States, based, no doubt, on his unfortunate experience with American publishers, and Miss Fuller must have shown concern lest her new friend should acquire a distorted notion of her country. "You have no cause for fearing that Harro Harring's sentiments could influence my opinion of the United States," Mazzini reassured her. "Harro Harring is no fit judge. His opinion are all derived from personal impulses. . . . As we must, I hope, agree about many more important things, so we do entirely agree about Harro" (*Appendix*, 6 : 507–9).

It has generally been assumed that Mazzini and Margaret Fuller first met at the Carlyles' and that Mazzini and George Lewes were both guests when Miss Fuller dined at the home of the Scottish sage. There is nothing in either Mazzini's writings or Miss Fuller's to support the assumption. On the contrary, considering the expressions of unbounded admiration she employed to describe him—"by far the most beauteous person I have seen," "he is beauteous as pure music"[8]—and considering the fact that she never mentioned him in connection with that dinner though she gave her impression of Lewes in detail, it is more plausible to assume that the Italian conspirator was not present on that occasion. They did spend one evening together with the Carlyles, however, and that was when Thomas and Jane Carlyle called on Miss Fuller before her departure. Mazzini was already there, and his presence roused Carlyle to an onslaught on progress, liberals, and their "rose-water imbecilities." Mazzini, after a few vain attempts to remonstrate, just sat there sadly under the sympathetic gaze of the two women, while Carlyle held forth on the theory that might makes right and on the necessity for unruly people to have yokes on their neck and "heroes" on their back.[9]

Mazzini's first impression of Miss Fuller was not overpowering. He mentioned casually in a letter to his mother that he had to "go and spend the evening at the house of an American writer, Miss Fuller, who is here for a few days" (30 : 256). Perhaps by that time he had perused her book, and knew that they agreed on "many important things"; but he did not know, what in his opinion was of greater importance, whether she possessed the enthusiasm and spirit of sacrifice necessary to transform her ideas into deeds. Her speech at the anniversary celebration of his Italian school dispelled that doubt.

For the previous four years Mazzini had held a sort of "open house" at his school on the anniversary of its foundation. He invited his friends, who in turn urged their own friends to attend, and usually a fairly large audience was on hand for the ceremony. Prizes were awarded to the best pupils, speeches were made, and some musical entertainment was contributed by outstanding singers or musicians who usually gladly consented to contribute their talents for the success of the occasion. After the ceremony a supper was served to the students, while the guests discussed the problems and needs of the school with Mazzini and left with him their contributions which, though modest, were usually sufficient to cover the expenses of operation for the following school year—rent, light, heat, and wages for a caretaker.

On November 10, at eight o'clock, after a day spent in packing for her imminent departure for Paris, Miss Fuller went to Greville Street. The room was crowded with three hundred guests. As usual there was a number of speeches, including one by Mazzini, and at the end Miss Fuller was invited to address the audience. In her

speech she remarked that there should be an international exchange, each country contributing what is best in their tradition:
the Germans, for instance, their simplicity, tireless industry, and
vast intellectual culture; the English, their mechanical ability and
their sense of honor; and the Italians, those arts that awaken the
love of the beautiful and the good. Italy, so beautiful in itself,
must be especially dear to poets and artists, and no one should be
indifferent to the efforts that country was making to free itself
from present degradation. The speaker was pleased to notice that
the Italians' innate love of beauty was revealed by the excellence of
the handwriting and drawing of the pupils of the school, and
concluded by urging her English friends present to help in the
teaching labors.[10]

Mazzini was quite pleased with the speech, which he punctu-
ated with vigorous approving nods. He knew now that, like him,
she believed that each country had a "mission" to accomplish, and
like him, she was not content with approving the good work done
by others, but felt it was every one's duty to lend a helping hand
in its performance. Three days later Mazzini wrote to his mother:
"The novelty of the ceremony was the speech made by an American lady I know, an eminent writer, well known here and in the
United States. She came and, requested by us to say a few words,
made a touching speech in which she said she would write about
what she saw, etc." (*30* : 269). This was a promise Miss Fuller
kept in her very first article from London to the *Tribune* (February
19, 1847), which was devoted to Mazzini, his ideas, and especially
his school which inspired her to a lyrical outburst.

Here these poor boys, picked up from the streets, are redeemed from
bondage and gross ignorance by the most patient and constant devotion of time and effort. What love and sincerity this demands from minds
capable of great thoughts, large plans, and rapid progress, only their
peers can comprehend; and as among the fishermen and poor people of
Judea were picked up those who have become to modern Europe a
leaven that leavens the whole mass, so may these poor Italian boys
become more efficacious as missionaries to their people than would an
Orphic poet at this period. . . . The whole evening gave a true and deep
pleasure, though tinged with sadness. We saw a planting of the Kingdom
of Heaven, though now no larger than a grain of mustard-seed, and
though perhaps none of those who watch the spot may live to see the
birds singing in its branches.[11]

Before leaving for Paris, Miss Fuller together with the Springs worked out a plan to smuggle Mazzini into Italy. They were going to Paris for a few weeks; Mazzini would join them there in disguise, and with an American passport they would secure for him would enter Italy as a member of their party.[12] The scheme looked perfectly feasible as they discussed it, perhaps in Greville Street after the celebration when they remained together until 1:30 in the morning. But after their departure he realized the difficulties the scheme involved. With a death sentence hanging over his head in Piedmont, and with the police of other Italian states only too willing to deliver him to the Piedmontese justice, a visit to Italy was too great a risk to run for mere personal pleasure. A visit to his mother "could not be ventured upon without making her frantic with terror," he explained on a different occasion (*Appendix*, 6 : 525). And finally, the enthusiasm aroused by the recent election of Pius IX indicated to him an awakening of national consciousness in Italy likely to lead, as it actually did lead shortly afterwards, to a revolutionary explosion, which required him to remain at his battle station—London. On December 24, Mazzini wrote to Miss Fuller enclosing letters of introduction to some Genoese friends and calling off the arrangements: "The scheme has unavoidably been protracted to some indefinite period. You guess it by my sending the introductory notes. I am bound here, not without a faint hope of revisiting my country in a different manner" (*Appendix*, 6 : 514).

Miss Fuller arrived in Paris on November 13 with letters to Lamberti. Mazzini recommended Miss Fuller, "a distinguished writer from the United States whom I greatly esteem and love," and her companions, "Mr. and Mrs. Spring, also American, very active in the cause of the poor negroes as well as any other cause founded on right and justice," and requested his friend to obtain for them the addresses of Madame Sand and Lamennais (*30* : 268). Marcus Spring called on Lamberti but unfortunately Spring spoke neither French nor Italian and Lamberti knew no English, and the interview resulted in an embarrassing conversational stalemate.[13] During the three months Miss Fuller spent in Paris, Mazzini heaped so many letters, messages, and errands for her upon poor, sickly Lamberti that the latter protested against that "unloading of all England and America" on him.[14] But in spite of his grumbling Lamberti called on Miss Fuller early in December and made several calls later on.[15] When she decided to prolong her stay in Paris beyond the planned few weeks visit and left the Grand Hotel Paris at Rue Richelieu for less expensive quarters on the outskirts of the city, he wrote resignedly to Mazzini: "Miss Fuller and the Springs will stay for two more months, and will go and live far away. And I, a confirmed boor disliking social life, will have to go and have tea with them some evening."[16]

Besides the messages he sent to Miss Fuller through Lamberti, Mazzini corresponded with her directly. It is unfortunate that only part of this correspondence is available. We have thirteen letters Mazzini wrote to Margaret Fuller, but he undoubtedly wrote more. Of the letters she wrote to him only one is extant, although we find in his correspondence reference to at least nine more. Mazzini followed the system, very wise in a conspirator, of destroying all letters he received soon after he answered them, preserving only those he considered of special importance, such as letters from Kossuth, George Sand, and a few others. To reconstruct a story from this one-sided correspondence is not unlike trying to catch the drift of a conversation by overhearing someone talking over the telephone. Fortunately in this instance Miss Fuller's letters to her friends and relatives and her articles in the *Tribune* help materially to round out the picture.

Three of the letters Mazzini wrote to Miss Fuller during her stay in Paris are extant. With the first, dated December 24, 1846, he enclosed four notes of introduction to friends in Italy—two in Genoa, one to Giuseppe Cornero in Turin, and one to Enrico Meyer in Florence—all full of high praise for the American writer and her companions. In the other two, dated January 17 and February 10, he requested Miss Fuller to contribute to the *People's Journal* some travel notes or anything else she might wish to write. Mazzini had been connected for some time with that liberal paper. A disagreement had lately developed between the editor, Saunders, and William Howitt which resulted in the latter's withdrawal from the paper to start his own *Howitt's Journal*, taking along with him a good number of collaborators. Mazzini hoped that in the reorganization of the paper he might be able to veer its policy more to the left. He was at that time attempting to organize—and he did so shortly thereafter—a "Peoples' International League" to arouse interest in the problems of oppressed nationalities, and he hoped to make the *Journal* a sort of unofficial organ of the League, the medium of expression "of the thought which in England and America dominates all souls noble and dedicated to the Future." But the immediate problem was to secure fresh funds and new writers. He urged Miss Fuller to help him herself, and expressed the hope that she might obtain the collaboration of Emerson also. The paper could not offer large remuneration—only thirty francs per page—but since its circulation exceeded twenty thousand copies, it offered an opportunity to air one's views to a rather wide circle (*Appendix*, *6*: 515–16, 518–19). Mazzini showed his eagerness to secure the collaboration of Miss Fuller by asking Lamberti (*32* : 53) and his mother (*32* : 71) to remind her of his request. Evidently he did not know, or had forgotten, that Miss Fuller had a contract with Horace Greely to write her "travel impressions" for the *Tribune*.

After a stay of three and one-half months in Paris, on February 25, 1847, Miss Fuller left for Italy. The crossing from Marseilles was long and miserable, "all one dull tormented dream," and the first sight of the magnificent marble palaces and garden of Genoa, seen in the cold blustering March wind, failed to charm her. "The weather was still so cold," she wrote home, "that I could not realize that I had actually touched those shores to which I had looked forward all my life, where it seemed that the heart would expand, and that the whole nature be turned to delight."[17] But the coldness of the weather was undoubtedly offset by the warm welcome she and the Springs received from Mazzini's family and friends. Since early in January Mazzini had been writing home of this visit, enclosing additional notes of introduction to people he wanted them to meet—Carolina Celesia, Fanny Balbi, Professor Pareto (*32* : 5, 19–20, 55–56, 71). He was pleased to hear that Miss Fuller and his mother had made a good impression on each other. "Your letter made me very happy," he wrote to his mother, "because of the report you give me of Miss Fuller, the affectionate ways she had with you, the cordial welcome she received, and everything. Only, I am sorry that her stay in Genoa was so short. . . . If by chance you write to her in Rome, express to her my gratitude for the affection she has shown you" (*32* : 76). A few days later he received a long letter from Miss Fuller, and wrote again to his mother: "She tells me a thousand things about you in ecstasy of admiration and sympathy; she speaks of Carolina, of whom she says, among other things, that she is the most beautiful woman she has so far seen on the continent; she speaks pleasantly of Miss Balbi; she did not see the Geologist [Pareto], because of her sudden departure. . . . She enclosed two leaves of lavender I think she picked from the window of the library. Two-thirds of the letter, however, are about you, with expressions that one almost cannot repeat, so highly laudatory are they!" (*32* : 92–93)

During that visit the two women must have spoken exclusively of the great agitator. Miss Fuller certainly expressed her great admiration and love for him, and the heart of Maria Mazzini went out to her. Seeing a woman intellectually brilliant, full of admiration and sympathy for her son, with the proper disparity of age between them, perhaps her mind, as mothers' minds often do, turned to thoughts of connubial possibilities, and she wrote to her son that she wished his American friend would settle in London and take care of him. Mazzini, who early in his exile had taken a vow of celibacy and could only offer fraternal affection to the admiring members of the other sex, felt embarrassed by the hardly veiled hint of his mother.

I tell you [he replied] not to desire that my American friend should reside in London to take care of me. Don't worry! If I were a man to yield and grow soft in the midst of Capuan delights, I would have all possible opportunities to do so: there are at least half a dozen young women, who contend each other the privilege of surrounding me with loving care. The Lord knows if I feel grateful to them, but I cannot afford to grow soft in the midst of their attentions. Sometime the excessive affection of these young friends of mine make me sad! Furthermore, if I yielded I would waste all my time with them (*32* : 93).

During her Italian tour in 1847, Miss Fuller and Mazzini had difficulty in maintaining the contact with each other they desired. One of her letters reached him unsealed by the Italian police (*32* : 163). Because of that he did not wish to reply by post, but he had difficulty in making other arrangements (*Appendix*, *6* : 526). Some tenuous contact was maintained through Mazzini's mother,[18] but during that Summer he knew only that she was somewhere in Switzerland, and, in spite of his efforts, he was not able to secure an address to reach her, as he was anxious to do (*32* : 230–31, 248, 316; *33* : 11).

It was only early in December on his return to London from a secret visit to the Continent that he found letters from Miss

Fuller, at that time in Rome where she had secretly and uncon-
ventionally married Marquis Ossoli. "Having seen that article in
the *Times* attacking me," he informed his mother, "she wrote an
article in the *People's Journal* in my praise, which I will send you"
(*33* : 142). Not in the *Times* but in *Galignani's Messenger* had Miss
Fuller read a reference to "the sanguinary schemes of Mazzini
and his associates," which that paper had quoted from the *Times*.
Miss Fuller wrote an indignant letter in which she stigmatized the
Galignani's Messenger as "a paper which, without talent to originate
anything good or bad, by a base instinct, delights to copy into its
columns whatever is adverse to the cause of progress." The writer
of the *Times*, she wrote, always showed "a love of falsehood or a
vindictive spirit." "To couple the epithet, sanguinary, with the
name of Mazzini," she continued, "would be simply absurd, as to
speak of the darkness of light."[19]

There was no correspondence between the two friends in 1848.
Mazzini's time and energy were completely taken up by political
activities. As soon as the revolution broke out he hastened to
Milan, where he strove to feed the patriotic fervor of the population and to enlist volunteers for the war against Austria in spite
of the hostility of the monarchical faction which watched his
activities with deep suspicion. After the defeat of Piedmont and
the reoccupation of Lombardy by Austria, he went to Switzerland
(August, 1848), and from there he tried unsuccesfully to revive
the revolutionary flame in Lombardy.

Miss Fuller at that time was going through a period of most
serious personal difficulties which she was reluctant to discuss
even with her most intimate friends. But she was more than ever
a loyal follower of Mazzini. Her correspondence to the *Tribune*
shows how in reporting the political events of that portentous
year, in passing judgment on the leading characters on the political
stage—King Charles Albert of Sardinia, the Pope, the King of
Naples, the Granduke of Tuscany, Mamiani, Gioberti, Pellegrino
Rossi—she consistently followed the "Mazzini line." The only
reservation she made on his program was that in his complete
absorption in the idea of political regeneration he neglected the
economic and social factors. "And yet Mazzini sees not all," she
wrote in her letter of April 19; "he aims at political emancipation;
but he sees not, perhaps would deny, the bearing of some events,
which even now begin to work their way. . . . I allude to that of

which the cry of Communism, the systems of Fourier, etc., are the forerunners."[20]

Personal contacts were re-established in the Spring of 1849. By that time the revolution had already been put down all over Italy, except in Venice, Rome, and Florence. In Florence it collapsed without a fight in April, and in Rome and Venice later, after a gallant but hopeless struggle. On February 8, after the flight of Pius IX from Rome, the Assembly decreed the end of the temporal power and the proclamation of the republic. On March 4, Mazzini, who had been previously elected to the Constituent Assembly, was made a Roman citizen, and on the following day he arrived in Rome. Two days earlier Miss Fuller had written to him a tender letter. To the melancholy thought he had expressed that, since he had not been able to live in his country, he had returned to die there, she replied: ". . . not so, dear Mazzini. You do not return to sleep under the sod of Italy, but to see your thoughts springing up all over her soil. The gardeners seem to me, in point of instinctive wisdom and deep thought, mostly incompetent to the care of the garden, but an idea like this, will be able to make use of any implements." And she went on to comfort him by reminding him that he should not feel discouraged if he was denied witnessing the full realization of his idea but should instead rejoice in the short advance made toward that fulfillment. "Men like you, appointed ministers must not be less earnest in their work, yet to the greatest, the day, the moment, is all their kingdom. God takes care of the increase."[21]

Three days after his arrival Mazzini went to call on Miss Fuller.

Last night, [she wrote to Marcus Spring] Mazzini came to see me.... I heard a ring; then somebody speak my name; the voice struck upon me at once. He looks more divine than ever, after all his new, strange sufferings. He asked after all of you. He stayed two hours, and we talked, though rapidly, of everything. He hopes to come often, but the crisis is tremendous, and all will come to him; since, if one can save Italy from her foes, inward and outward, it will be he. But he is very doubtful whether this will be possible; the foes are too many, too strong, too subtle. Yet Heaven helps sometime. I only grieve I cannot aid him; freely would I give my life to aid him.... I fear that it is in reserve for him, to survive defeat. True, he can never be utterly defeated; but to see Italy bleeding, prostrate once more, will be very dreadful for him.... All this I write to you, because you said, when I was suffering at leaving Mazzini, "You will meet him in Heaven." This I believe will be, despite all my faults.[22]

It is well known that Margaret Fuller took an active part in the defense of the Roman republic. On May 30, 1849, she was appointed superintendent of the hospital *Fate-bene-fratelli*, and throughout the period of the siege she spent most of her time caring for the wounded, while her husband, Marquis Ossoli, fought in the defense of the city as captain of the militia. Her letters to the *Tribune*, as well as her personal letters to her family and friends, show how keenly she felt the tragedy of the infant Roman republic doomed to fall under the blows of a sister republic, France, in coalition with Naples, Spain, and Austria, the most reactionary monarchies in Europe. Her admiration for Mazzini, for the way he was meeting the greatest test of his life, was unbounded. At the height of the siege (June 10) she wrote to Emerson:

Speaking of the republic you say, "Do you not wish Italy had a great man?" Mazzini is a great man. In mind a great, poetic statesman; in heart, a lover; in action, decisive and full of resources as Caesar. Dearly I love Mazzini. He came in, just as I had finished the first letter to you. His soft radiant look makes melancholy music in my soul; it consecrates my present life, that, like the Magdalen, I may, at the important hour, shed the consecrated ointment on his head.[23]

Mazzini must have found comfort in the love and loyalty of this faithful disciple. In a note (June 9) written evidently in reply to a complaint of neglect he told her:

Will you be a woman and forgive? I will deserve to be forgiven; could you spend a whole day near me, you would wonder not at my being silent with those I love, but at my living.... Everything from the detail of a soldier arrested at St. Angelo to the defense, from a quarrel between two officers to a dissenting between two generals comes down to me. I scarcely even write a few words to my mother. Should the thing last long there is no human strength or will that can resist.... I have often been thinking of you, the only thing that I can do. Keep faithful and trustful; pray for Rome and Italy; it is centered here (*Appendix*, 6 : 537–39).

As the pressure of the besieging armies increased, defeatist rumors began to circulate in Rome, one of which was that St. Peter's church had been mined by the republicans. The aim of the rumor obviously was to spread concern and resentment among the people who were strongly attached to their "cupolone." The rumor must have found some credence, because Miss Fuller wrote to Mazzini to inquire about it, to the pained surprise of the Triumvir.

It is written that none will trust me [he replied]; you too! Can you believe for a single moment such nonsense as that of St. Peter being mined, whilst I am here? Have I proven a Vandal, or a man of '93? Is there a Frenchwoman here who has been molested?... My soul is full of grief and bitterness, and still I have never for a moment yielded to reactionary feelings. Let people talk about St. Peter; it may be of some use, but depend upon a friendly word: no one has seen the mines; no one will ever see them! I repeat, whilst I am here. Write every time you like to do so. Do not punish me for my not being able to write to my friends (*Appendix*, 6 : 539–41).

When the defense of the Roman republic was no longer possible the Assembly voted to surrender, and the Triumvirs resigned in protest. Mazzini asked Margaret's help to secure American passports for the seriously compromised popular leader, Angelo Brunetti (Ciceruacchio), and his thirteen-year-old son, who were afraid of the revenge of the Papal government, and possibly one for himself (*Appendix*, 6 : 542–44). Perhaps through Miss Fuller, who was a personal friend of the American Minister Lewis Cass, Jr., American passports were released to Ciceruacchio and his son, Mazzini, and Avezzana, and an American corvette was placed at the disposal of Garibaldi at Civitavecchia to facilitate his flight. Unfortunately, except for Avezzana, who shortly afterwards returned to New York and was received enthusiastically by the Italians there,[24] the others either did not make use of or get any protection from the generous help of the American Ambassador. Ciceruacchio and his son were captured and shot by the Austrians; Garibaldi, after his heroic but futile attempt to reach Venice with the remnants of his army to continue the fight there, was barely able to find sanctuary into Piedmontese territory; and Mazzini had to effect his escape without any documents, because his American passport lacked the visa of the French authorities. Just before leaving he inquired unsuccessfully of Miss Fuller if she knew of any English or American party going to Switzerland that he could join so that his American passport would look more authentic (*Appendix*, 6 : 544–46).

After Rome was occupied by the French troops, both Mazzini and Miss Fuller left the city, Mazzini to go to Switzerland and eventually back to London, Miss Fuller to go first to Rieti in the Umbrian hills and then to Florence, whence she departed the following year for her ill-fated return journey to America. Before leaving she paid her last tribute of devotion to Mazzini in a letter to her brother-in-law, W. C. Channing.

I did not see Mazzini, the last two weeks of the Republic. When the French entered, he walked about the streets, to see how people bore themselves, and then went to the house of a friend. ... I found him. ... Mazzini had suffered millions more than I could; he had borne his fearful responsibility; he had let his dearest friends perish; he had passed all those nights without sleep; in two months, he had grown old; all the vital juices seemed exhausted; his eyes were all bloodshot; his skin orange; flesh he had none; his hair was mixed with white; his hand was painful to the touch; but he never flinched, never quailed; had protested in the last hour against the surrender; sweet and calm, but full of a more fiery purpose than ever; in him I revered the hero, and owned myself not of that mould.[25]

During her stay in Florence Miss Fuller collected the materials for her book on the ephemeral Roman republic, and perhaps actually wrote it. Just before her return to America she had tried to make arrangements for its publication both in England and America. At the time of her tragic shipwreck near the shore of New Jersey, her friends who knew of the book hoped and tried to recover the manuscript but without success.[26] Perhaps the book that many of her friends expected to be her masterpiece was lost in the shipwreck, perhaps it was destroyed by the "wreckers" who robbed the baggage washed ashore by the storm. Garibaldi, who was in America at the time, related that he heard it had been destroyed by a Catholic priest.[27] Later, Hawthorne reported on the assertion of Mozier, the American sculptor in Rome, that the book had never been written and that "the *History of the Roman Revolution*, about which there was so much lamentation in the belief that it had been lost with her, never had any existence."[28]

The year after her death, her friends—Emerson among them—decided to publish a selection of her writings as a sort of memorial to her. They wrote to the eminent people she had known in Europe and requested literary contributions. Mazzini was asked by Emerson for an account of her Italian years, but his reply never reached its destination. He was again requested through James Russell Lowell, but again his contribution failed to arrive. "Spite of all Mazzini did not write. I feared he would not, for to tell the truth—Guy Fawkes was too busy with his lanthorn and matches to be writing letters," reported Lowell to Emerson[29] with a malicious reference to the preparations Mazzini was making with Kossuth for the Milanese revolt of 1853.

With the death of Margaret Fuller, Mazzini not only lost a friend and kindred spirit but also a gifted writer who could have, and certainly would have, done much to advance in America his ideas on the regeneration of Italy. She was a champion of his cause he sorely missed, especially when American public opinion in the fifties veered toward the program of the Savoy monarchy. Margaret Fuller, during the last four years of her life, the years in which, to use the expression of Harriet Martineau, she was transformed "from the dreaming and haughty pedant into the true woman,"[30] was fully, almost exclusively under the influence of Mazzini, who inspired in her great enthusiasm and devotion for his ideal. Only her untimely death prevented her from keeping the promise she made in a letter to Emerson: "There is one, Mazzini, who understands thee well—who knew thee no less when an object of popular fear than now of idolatry—and who, if the pen be not held too feebly, will help posterity to know thee too."[31]

Chapter V

MAZZINI AND THE AMERICAN OFFICIALS IN ROME

THE ELECTION of Pius IX aroused much enthusiasm among liberals inside and out of Italy. Many Italians deluded themselves with the wishful thought that the new, kindly, and humane ruler of the Papal states would turn into an incarnation of Gioberti's mythical religious leader and would somehow bring about the the political regeneration of Italy. Americans, irrespective of their religious faith, also took great interest in the "liberal" Pope, an interest which, in the words of Horace Greely, "ripened into sympathy and unmeasured admiration." Although a few thoughtful writers foresaw the difficulties the Pope was bound to encounter, the American press was unanimous in its praise of the mild reforms he had granted his people. Between the end of 1847 and the beginning of 1848, mass meetings were held in a number of American cities. Leading political figures participated in them, and resolutions were passed expressing the earnest sympathy of the American people for the enlightened policy of the new Pope. American public opinion expressed itself strongly also in favor of the establishment of regular diplomatic relations with the Papal states, and, in response to that demand, President Polk, in his message to Congress of December 7, 1847, recommended that such a step be taken for political as well as economic reasons. In March, 1848, Congress passed the necessary appropriations, and Dr. Jacob L. Martin, secretary of the American embassy in Paris, was appointed chargé d'affaires to the Papal court.

Events meanwhile had moved rapidly in the rest of Italy. Early in 1848, all the Italian native rulers had been forced by rebellion or threat of rebellion to grant constitutional governments to their people. The King of Naples granted a constitution on January 29, the King of Sardinia on February 7, and the Granduke of Tuscany on February 17. The French revolution on February 24 and the fall and flight of Metternich on March 13 touched off the revolutionary explosion in Milan and Venice where the people drove the Austrian garrisons out and established provisional governments. By the end of March, 1848, the revolution had triumphed all over Italy.

But at the very moment when complete victory seemed assured, a tug of war developed between the monarchists and the republicans for control of the movement. The republicans tried to enlist the help of the American chargé d'affaires for their cause. On May 1, Dr. Martin, at that time still in Paris, reported to the State Department that several agents from the Republican party in Milan and Venice had urged him to show his sympathy for their cause by stopping at Milan on his way to his residence in Rome so that the prestige of an American representative could be used to further the republican propaganda in those cities. The request was refused.[1] Within a few months the liberal movement collapsed. The King of Sardinia was defeated on the battlefield, and Lombardy and most of the Venetian provinces were reoccupied by the Austrians. The King of Naples withdrew the constitution, and re-established the absolute government. The Pope and the Granduke of Tuscany, failing in their attempt to follow his example, fled their states and sought the protection of Naples and Austria, respectively. By the end of 1848, the only liberal regimes still in existence in Italy were the Kingdom of Sardinia and the precarious provisional governments of Rome, Venice, and Tuscany, against which Austria was preparing to take action.

The American Ambassador to the Papal states did not reach Rome until August 3, 1848, and died there suddenly on the twenty-sixth of the same month, before he could present his credentials to the Papal court. The American Legation remained vacant until the appointment of the new chargé d'affaires, Lewis Cass, Jr., several months later. During this vacancy, consul Nicholas Brown, a militant liberal, sent to the State Department glowing accounts of the activities of the liberal government in Rome. When the Constituent Assembly decreed the end of the temporal power and the proclamation of the republic, Brown attended the ceremony in his consular uniform and addressed congratulatory notes to Monsignor Muzzarelli, President of the Council of Ministers, and Signor

Rusconi, Minister of Foreign Affairs, expressing his conviction that soon the American government would grant official recognition to the newly born sister republic. He strongly urged in his dispatches that the American government follow such a course.

I have endeavored throughout the course of my remarks [he wrote in his report of March 27] to give a faithful picture of the occurrences here, and show the Roman revolution with its causes and consequences in their true light. I felt this the more incumbent on me as a very large proportion of the European press, eager to gain or preserve the encouragement & support of the aristocratic & monarchical factions, have either substituted fictions for facts, or compelled their readers to view those truths which could not be concealed, through a confusing and distorting medium. To this circumstance, conjointly with a conscientiously erroneous, or hypocritically feigned apprehension that the interests of our Holy Religion would suffer serious injury by the sacrifice of the pope's temporal power: to these causes, I say, is alone owing the non recognition of the Roman Republic by the whole world, or the far greater portion of it. Yet all the circumstances connected with the establishment of the republic plead loudly, invincibly for her recognition.[2]

And on April 30, he repeated:

If in my previous communications I concluded a faithful however feeble picture of the events which had occurred in the Roman State, & the feelings which animated its inhabitants, by urging upon our government the justice and propriety of an immediate recognition of the infant republic, I little anticipated so speedy, so peremptory a justification of all I advanced.[3]

At length Brown tired of recommending a course of action which his superiors had decided not to follow at the time, and on May 19, just before he resigned (or was recalled) he wrote: "If the recognition of this Republic, by her great trans-atlantic sister has not yet taken place, this omission (so I deem it) can certainly not be laid to my charge; and, under existing circumstances, as any further insisting on this point would be superfluous, & might be thought presumptuous, I shall say no more."[4]

And indeed, the instructions that James Buchanan had sent to Lewis Cass, Jr. on February 16 excluded categorically the possibility of the recognition of the Roman republic. The State Department felt that although the established policy of the United States had been, and still was, to grant recognition to any government irrespective of its origin so long as it enjoyed popular support, this policy could not be followed in the case of the Roman republic, because the difficulties surrounding that regime made most unlikely the eventuality of its survival. Cass was directed to maintain a position of neutrality. He proceeded to Rome, the seat of the Republican government, rather than to Gaeta, the Papal court in exile, but refrained from presenting his credentials to the Republican government.

On his arrival in Rome, Cass was besieged by both friends and foes of the republic, all urging him to act according to their preferences. The leaders of the republic, Mazzini among them, solicited him to present his credentials and establish diplomatic relations, hoping thus to break the diplomatic boycott established against them by the European chancelleries. Dinners and seats at the opera were offered to him, but he declined. The foes of the republic exerted themselves to prevent such a recognition. Two diplomats accredited to the Papal court who had followed the Pope at Gaeta—the Minister of Prussia and the Secretary of the French legation—returned to Rome on April 17 and paid Cass a call, ostensibly a courtesy call, to dissuade him from presenting his credentials. The powers, they assured him, were certain to intervene to put down the revolutionary spirit which under the guise and name of democracy was spreading so much evil, and intervention spelled the certain doom of the republic and the speedy restoration of the Papal rule.

Cass himself at first shared these doubts about the stability of the Roman republic. But shortly after his arrival he began to revise some of his opinions. Contrary to the erroneous idea broadcast in America by the Catholic press—that only a few rabid radicals were opposed to the Papal rule—he found to his surprise that a great many people of education, position, and means—the people, in short, who constitute the core of the conservative group everywhere—expressed to him a vehement opposition to the Papal rule and assured him that a re-establishment of the old regime might determine them to leave the country. Another source of surprise was the satisfactory way the Republican administration was working in spite of the innumerable difficulties they had to meet.

When France decided to intervene in behalf of the Pope, the hopelessness of the situation became apparent to all, and Cass felt certain that the Romans would not put up a futile resistance. "The Romans of the present day," he reported in one of his dispatches," are not disposed to strike, even for honor and for right, without very good prospect of success." But the Romans surprised him once again. A few days later the first attack of the French expeditionary force was repulsed with heavy losses, and Cass reported that the Romans, "contrary to all expectations . . . made a brave and gallant resistance"; that the appearance of the invader had united all the people, even those of tepid republicanism, in the resolve to fight for their independence; that in the city everbody was bearing the sacrifices imposed by the critical situation "with cheerfulness and alacrity," while from the country offers of men and money for the defense of the capital were hourly pouring in. Most of the American colony had remained in the city and was sharing the popular enthusiasm for the republic, to which it had made so many offers of assistance and financial contributions that on different occasions the Assembly had passed resolutions expressing the nation's gratitude to the American citizens.

The popular fervor must have been infectious. The admiring tone of the subsequent dispatches Cass wrote detailing the courage and the single-mindedness of the defenders of Rome shows that he too had fallen under its spell. On May 23 he reported as follows:

While external dangers are . . . augmenting, the unanimity of the people in support of the government appears to advance proportionably. The various factions, which were in existence a few weeks previously, have coalesced into one attitude, that of the defense of the republic; and expressions of patriotism and resolutions to suffer to the last extremity, is the only language heard in the streets. In Rome's best days, when the Capitol was menaced by a foreign foe, no better or braver spirit was ever manifested, than the same scenes now exhibit. To meet the extraordinary expenses of the government, not a few citizens, embracing every condition, have placed their entire fortunes, unreservedly, at the disposal of the Ministry. And in the conduct of this nature the women have borne their part—their contribution consisting of jewelry and ornaments—gold, silver, and precious stones—some of which are reported to be of enormous value. . . . It is difficult to remain an indifferent spectator of such a struggle. . . . To our countrymen here, several of whom are known to you as persons of distinction and fortune, it is a subject of some regret, that our government has not deemed it advisable to recognize at once the new republic. . . . Without entering into political considerations, yielding to natural feelings springing from education and associations, they have evinced their partiality for the republican cause, by contributing pecuniary aid to the Ministry, since the commencement of military operations; and so gratefully is this conduct regarded, that the Assembly have passed a resolution, declaring American citizens to be under the immediate protection of the State, their person inviolable, and that a military commission will instantly judge the first act of violence of which they may complain.[5]

American public opinion meanwhile was expressing itself strongly in favor of the immediate recognition of the Roman republic. A precedent had been established the year before when the French republic was recognized without delay. Lewis Cass, Jr. was criticized for his failure to present his credentials. It was not generally known, evidently, that his instructions precluded such an action on his part. The pressure at home, combined with the increasingly favorable reports the State Department was receiving from Cass, determined the administration to revise the instructions to the chargé d'affaires and give him discretionary powers to present his credentials to any Roman government which in his opinion had the necessary prerequisites of stability and popular support to warrant such an action.

It would appear . . . that the affairs of the Papal States have become more and more complicated and entangled. It has always been the policy and practice of the United States to acknowledge new governments; and the delay in recognizing that of Rome, has arisen entirely from the opinion (which may be an erroneous one) that it did not possess the proper elements of stability.

The President, however, is unwilling to keep you bound by instructions too stringent for the occasion, and thereby, to prevent you from doing that, at the proper time, which ought to be done; whether in reference to the government now in apparent authority, or to any other which may be substituted for it, possessing the necessary requisite of stability. Of the exact nature of the circumstance, and of the conditions of the affairs, which would warrant and even make it desirable, as well as proper, that such a step should be taken, we cannot so well nor so properly judge, at this distance, as you may, who are on the spot. But, after duly weighing the matter, the President has directed me to say, that he leaves it entirely to your discretion to present, whenever you shall deem it best, your letter of Credence to the Minister of Foreign Relations of the Provisional Government; or to withhold it some time longer, if the latter course should seem to your judgment preferable.

Although we have not yet learned that the Provisional Government has received the recognition of any other government, we certainly do not desire to be behind any in this Act of Grace and Courtesy.[6]

Unfortunately these instructions were dated June 25, only a few days before the fall of the Roman republic, and were received by Cass long after the French army had entered Rome and re-established the Papal rule. The Washington correspondent of the *New York Herald* reported the news of the enlarged instructions on July 3,[7] which, by an ironical coincidence, was the very day the Constituent Assembly was forcibly disbanded by the French troops after it had, as a sort of last will and testament, officially enacted the new republican constitution.

The Roman republic remained an object of sympathy long after it had ceased to exist. A London correspondent of the *New York Herald* argued that official recognition on the part of the United States might have saved the republican governments in Rome and in Hungary. The same thesis was maintained by Kossuth later on during his American tour. In 1855, the Democratic societies of New York held a mass meeting in the Broadway Tabernacle to commemorate the sixth anniversary of the foundation of the Roman republic. At the meeting the re-establishment of the Papal rule by foreign bayonets was decried and the rebirth of the republic in Italy was presaged.[8] The American press strongly criticized the French intervention, and the motives of Louis Napoleon were viewed prophetically as the first step toward the destruction of the republic in France. Mass meetings were held in several American cities in the Summer of 1849 at which resolutions were passed stigmatizing Louis Napoleon as the "Judas Iscariot of liberty" and the "Benedict Arnold of the old world," who had "earned for himself a page in history worthy of being placed in the most bloody and cruel annals of the past," and whose crushing of the Roman Republic was "an act of turpitude so base that the stain can never be effaced."[9]

During his leadership of the Roman republic Mazzini was for the first time in contact with American officials, notably consul Nicholas Brown and chargé d'affaires Lewis Cass, Jr. Of the two, Mazzini much preferred Brown. His impulsiveness and his openly proclaimed sympathy for the Roman republic endeared him to Mazzini, who contrasted his behavior with that of Cass, whose sincere sympathy for the Italian cause was necessarily concealed under the formalities of diplomatic correctness. "Cass, the chargé d'affaires of the Republic to us," Mazzini wrote to Foresti, "behaved very badly; if he had recognized us, as he ought to have, it would have helped us greatly. Brown, the American consul in Rome, conducted himself very well" (*42* : 17).

After leaving Rome, Brown kept in touch with Mazzini for several years. He visited Mazzini in Switzerland in September, 1849, and on his way back to Italy he stopped at Genoa to visit with Mazzini's mother (*42* : 42) who gave him a cordial reception (*42* : 48). The following year he informed Mazzini that an American newspaper had exhumed the rumor of the mining of the Vatican which had been circulated in Rome during the siege. "The former American consul in Rome," he wrote again to Foresti, "a friend of mine and an enthusiastic supporter of ours, writes that some American paper has brought out the accusation that we intended to blow up the Vatican, and insinuated that Cass persuaded us not to do it. He wants us to refute it. The accusation is absurd! Why don't Avezzana or Filopanti deny it, appealing publicly to Cass, Jr.? Lukewarm as he was, he knew me well, and should feel honor bound to deny it himself" (*44* : 167). In 1853, while consul at Constantinople, Brown acted as liaison between Italian and Hungarian patriots (*50* : 204). Three years later he wrote to Mazzini for details on the death of Ugo Bassi, the patriotic priest executed by the Austrians in Bologna in 1849, whose name figured quite prominently in the American press in 1853 on the occasion of the visit to America of Monsignor Bedini, Papal Nuncio at the Brazilian court. "Brown asks me," Mazzini wrote to Dall'Ongaro, "not a few lines but a complete report, with names and dates, on the Bassi affair. I know the facts only vaguely. Have you ever written a complete report on it? If so, send it to me immediately; I will translate into English and sign it. Take care, however, that your eargerness to harm those traitors does not lead to exaggerations. Even against my enemies I have never in my life signed anything I did not believe true" (*57* : 121). Perhaps it was also Brown who sent Mazzini "an urgent request . . . from America" for "news, references, historical data on the life and miracles (that is, persecution of liberals) of Monsignor Bedini" (*57* : 260–61) which Mazzini passed on to Count Luigi Pianciani, a Roman liberal in exile in London, who presumably had more information on that subject.

Mrs. Brown shared her husband's enthusiasm for liberal ideas, as well as his customary lack of caution. With her husband she visited Mazzini in Switzerland, where he gave her a letter of introduction to an unidentified prominent French liberal, perhaps Lamennais (*Appendix, 4 : 82*). The following year she was expelled from Naples because of her association with people suspected of liberalism. Lewis Cass, Jr., obviously amused by her misadventure, informed Margaret Fuller: "Have you heard that Mrs. Brown, our *quondam* Consuless, has been ordered to leave Naples? It appears she has been making herself very conspicuous there, by assembling around her a few rather 'mauvais sujets,' forgetting that she no longer possesses inviolability of domicile, and the authorities, in the most peremptory manner, compelled her to leave."[10]

Cass, on the other hand, was never forgiven by Mazzini for his failure to recognize the Roman republic. As soon as Cass reached Rome, Brown urged him to recommend immediate recognition, but he refused because he thought that the "government would not last a week; that it would fall to pieces of itself, as he had been told by the best authorities in England."[11] Perhaps Brown had in mind these "best authorities in England," when he wrote in his report of March 7, prepared shortly after the arrival of Cass, that only reactionaries were in favor of the re-establishment of the Papal rule.

Possibly even England might complacently look on. Her proud aristocracy, conscious that their power exists only through the perpetuation of bigotry & prejudice, dread that a republic in Europe, happy and flourishing, should confirm, by another example, the great truth our own stupendous Republic is daily and practically impressing upon the subject of Queen Victoria. Even the merchants of that Kingdom, eager to amass that wealth which shall, some day, enable them or their descendants, to enter the hallowed precincts of the courtly circle, will, too many of them, dream of that peace, only however to be purchased at the expense of the happiness, etc., well being of their fellow creatures, which will enable them to lay Italy under contribution.[12]

Cass, however, did change his opinion after he witnessed the gallant defense of the Romans. His dispatches to the State Department became increasingly more favorable as time went on, though never as partisan and oratorical as Brown's reports. A dispatch he wrote on August 14 after the fall of the republic contains as forceful an indictment of the Papal rule and as eloquent a defense of the fallen republic as Mazzini himself could have penned.

The overthrow of the republican party, not only in Rome, but throughout Italy, and the entire prostration of the liberal cause as a barrier against the inroad of despotic power, must now be taken as a fact. The late issue was not, as the European press has so constantly insinuated, between anarchy and order; it was between constitutional, representative government, and the most benumbing despotism, whose rule, protracted through a few more years, at the cost of debt, poverty, ignorance, and the paralyzation of all improvement, must again result in a universal uproar, as the natural fruit of arbitrary misgovernment. When this Revolution is set before us in the exact proportion with which history will adjust it, it will be seen that, in the principle involved, something more was at stake than the independence of Rome, or the ascendency of the Triumvirate; viz. the peace, the liberties, progress and civilization of Europe against the very existence of irresponsible and despotic government.[13]

After the French occupation of Rome, Cass aided the most compromised of the leaders to flee the city. He issued passports to Mazzini, Avezzana, Brunetti and his son, the Prince of Canino, and perhaps to others. For Mazzini he also wrote a letter of introduction and recommendation to H. S. Paisily, American consul at Genoa, couched in the most complimentary terms for the Italian agitator, "a man of great integrity of character, and of most extensive intellectual acquirements," whose "whole life has been devoted to the cause of liberty and independence" (*40* : 212–13).

When the story of the issuance of those passports was published in the American press, Cass denied it. He claimed, in a dispatch to the State Department, that consul Brown, together with other foreign consuls, had released a number of passports to "Italians whose lives were in jeopardy" but without representing them as American citizens and that he personally "gave open letters to four individuals, among whom were Mazzini, one of the Triumvirate, and Charles Bonaparte, Prince of Canino," in which the kind offices of American consuls at some Mediterranean ports were requested in their behalf.[14] Mazzini heard of this denial several years later and heatedly refuted it. "Cass lies," he wrote to a friend. "I had a passport from him, through poor Miss Fuller's unrequested exertions, I believe; I had it when I was already in

Civitavecchia, that is, after having been seven or eight days in Rome, putting all my friends in despair, and walking leisurely through the streets, when everybody had left. The passport reached me without any visa for France. I sent it back" (*57* : 116–17).

The truth of the matter is that Mazzini and Avezzana were given passports under the assumed names of George Moore (Mazzini) and Everett (Avezzana), under names, that is, that could easily be taken for American. If Mazzini received his passport while in Civitavecchia, he could not have received it from Brown who had already left Rome. But one cannot help feeling that Mazzini's outburst against Cass, although done only in a private letter, was certainly ungracious and that he should have remembered that even if Cass had lied he had done so in connection with an attempt to save his life and that of his friends. It is likely that Mazzini's resentment against Cass was increased by the tokens of consideration the latter received from the Papal government as the representative of the United States, which Mazzini must have mistaken as an indication of Cass's sympathy for the reactionary cause.

Because of this misunderstanding Mazzini even tried to have him recalled from his post. This happened when Kossuth had just returned from his triumphal tour of America, where he had made contacts with leading political personalities. Mazzini, evidently ignorant of the high standing Senator Cass, father of the chargé d'affaires, had in the Democratic party and in the administration, must have written to Kossuth (the letter is not extant) that he wished to have Lewis Cass recalled from his post. Kossuth replied:

As for Cass, I am sorry, but I do not think he can be recalled, out of consideration for his father. But give me your advice as to what you wish he should receive in the way of instructions, and, if the thing is possible, it shall be done. We could also have his father write to him a few words of advice, which would be worth reams of instructions. ... In general you would do well to prepare a note on what sort of instructions you would like for American agents in Italy. I have done so in general and on principle, on all that I believed would interest you, but you may have some special wishes of which I am ignorant. I could have them brought to the attention of the Secretary of State.[15]

It is a curious commentary on this misunderstanding that while Mazzini was attempting to have Cass removed because of his presumed sympathy with the reaction the American diplomat used his influence to have thirteen political prisoners released from the Roman prisons and personally paid three thousand dollars for their passage to California.[16]

Another American official in Rome who roused the wrath of Mazzini was Edwin C. Cushman, the nephew of the famous American actress, Charlotte Cushman, who was consul at Rome from 1865 to 1869 and who also for the last two years of service was in charge of the American Legation. When Garibaldi invaded the Papal states in 1867, Cushman went along with the Papal troops as a self-appointed observer. He was present at, and participated in, a skirmish between the Papal troops and Garibaldi's legionaries, and was slightly wounded in the engagement. The undiplomatic conduct of Cushman was reported to Secretary of State Seward by Richard Rothwell, an English artist residing in Rome, and by Jos. J. Lewis from Naples. Rothwell, in a shocked and indignant letter, charged that Cushman "armed with his rifle joined the party who call themselves the 'Modern Crusaders,' and are known here as Zouaves"; that "for two days this American did Godly service with his friends the Zouaves in mortal conflict against the Italians whose nobility of soul has aroused them to seek a Nationality"; and that he "returned to Rome . . . proudly boasting of the wound he had received," which "unfortunately was not 'wide as a church door' but enough to mark his infamy and to cast a stigma on the proud republic of America."[17]

This letter was sent to Cushman by Seward with a request for explanation. Cushman denied that he had joined the Zouaves "with his rifle," asserting that he had, with the permission of the commanding general, accompanied a column as a spectator in order to obtain reliable information to transmit to the Department. During a skirmish an officer he was with fell wounded, and while he was trying to assist him he himself came under fire and picked up a gun in self-defense. Since Cushman's explanation confirmed the main points of the accusation, the Department subjected him to an official reprimand.

The American friends of the European republicans were not satisfied with this issue of the question, and tried to gather additional proofs of Cushman's unfitness for his office in order to have him removed. For this purpose they wrote to Mazzini, who in turn requested Andrea Giannelli in Florence for assistance in the matter.

A certain Cushman, American Consul or Agent in Rome, during the last events conducted himself as a papist: he left the city with the Zouaves, and fired on our legions. He was reprimanded by Seward, but we are not satisfied. My American friends and I want him dismissed. For this purpose they need information on his conduct before the action, exact data that prove that he was always opposed to us, etc. Perhaps it will be difficult to gather them; nevertheless you should write to Rome, tell our friends to do whatever they can, and write me a letter on the subject that I can copy or quote. It is a thing unimportant in itself, but it would be a lesson to those agents of the United States who disregard their instructions (*87* : 29–30).

Giannelli's reply is not extant, but it is likely that Mazzini did receive from him some additional charges to transmit to his friends in America, because shortly after Seward wrote to Cushman that some American residents in Rome were complaining he was neglecting his regular consular duties, because of his interest in politics. This Cushman denied and alleged that his enemies, encouraged by the reprimand he had previously suffered, were trying to bring him into further disfavor with the Department of State. Seward must have accepted the explanation, because Cushman remained at his post for another year,[18] until shortly before the end of the Papal regime.

CHAPTER VI

THE AMERICAN TOUR OF LOUIS KOSSUTH

AFTER THE FALL of the Roman republic, Mazzini took refuge in Switzerland, where he remained for over a year under the name of William Emerson. Undaunted by the catastrophe, he felt certain that the defeat suffered by his party all over Europe was only a temporary setback, a Pyrrhic victory for the enemy, and that a fresh opportunity to renew the fight would soon occur, perhaps within months. He was convinced that the first spark for the new conflagration would come again from France. Consequently he immediately set himself to pick up and reweave the threads of his organization which had been broken up and scattered by the recent political and military events. Like his previous organizations, this, too, was centered in a journal, the *Italia del Popolo* (the People's Italy) whose name epitomized its program. The unification of Italy was to be achieved by the people without the aid of the princes—aid which had so hopefully and mistakenly been sought by the naive enthusiasts of 1848 and which had been not the least cause of the failure of the movement.

One of the first leaders he contacted was Foresti, who was urged to reorganize the party among the Italians and to obtain subscriptions for the journal among Italians and sympathetic Americans. Believing that the Roman republic was the legally constituted government of the Papal states—the one sanctioned by popular suffrage—and that its officials, though prevented from exercising their functions by a foreign army of occupation, were still the representatives of the country, Mazzini felt that, as a "government in exile," the party had the right to appoint delegates and representatives abroad. Accordingly, Foresti was appointed on January 20, 1850, Delegate of the Triumvirate in America.

By these presents Citizen Felice Foresti is appointed Delegate of the Triumvirate, and charged with the following mission: 1. To promote and help with general regulations and advices, the organization of patriotic Italians scattered throughout the United States—under the flag of the *Italia del Popolo*. 2. To receive every two months from the centers of the Association already established or to be established in the great American division, the list of members and their monthly dues, one-third of which is to be sent to the Triumvirate for its general expenses. 3. To hasten the formation of deposits of arms and war material for the war of independence. 4. To direct a propaganda aiming at establishing solid and active sympathies for the Italian cause among the people of the United States. 5. To correspond with the Triumvirate about everything that may concern the progress of said cause, and the mission entrusted with the present delegation.

[Signed] Gius. Mazzini, A. Saffi, M. Montecchi (*40* : 250–1)

In the course of 1850, Mazzini's plan of reorganization was broadened into an attempt to bind together all the revolutionary forces in Europe. The revolution of 1848, by fortuitous coördination spread rapidly all over the Continent, taking the governments by surprise and quickly achieving its initial victory. But as soon as the conservative forces recovered from the initial shock, they mustered their forces and moved in concert against the various national movements which, being unconnected, fell one by one under the combined attack. The lessons the liberals had to learn from the debacle were (1) the need to coördinate their efforts so that an outbreak anywhere could count on the support of fellow revolutionists everywhere on the Continent and (2) the need to counterbalance the "Holy Alliance of the Despots" with a "Holy Alliance of the Peoples" which could count on the sympathy, perhaps the support, of the free countries—England and America.

This "Holy Alliance of the Peoples" was the goal of the organization of European Democracy, which was established along lines similar to the "Young Europe" of the early and middle thirties but set up for revolutionary action rather than for propaganda work. The directing body was the Central European Committee, consisting of one member from each of the nationalities represented. Underneath it were the various national committees in charge of the secret societies in their own home lands and of the organization of the patriots residing abroad. And finally, at the base were the various local committees, which for the Italians were established in many Italian centers and in numerous cities abroad, such as Paris, Geneva, Lugano, Malta, Tunis, Barcellona, Constantinople, Athens, New York, and New Orleans. The task of these local committees was to organize the patriots, collect funds, and arouse sympathy for their cause among the natives of the various countries in which they resided.

The scheme of the organization was outlined by Mazzini to Foresti toward the end of 1850. The Central European Committee set up in London included Ledru-Rollin for France, Mazzini for Italy, Darasz for Poland, Ruge for Germany, Golesco for Roumania, Klapka for Hungary, and "others who will be revealed gradually." The Italian National Committee, also residing in London, consisted of Mazzini and five other patriots from various regions of Italy. A number of local committees, Mazzini assured the Italian national Committee, had also been established already. "Now it is up to you," Mazzini continued.

It is urgent that you, Avezzana, and Filopanti should formally constitute the Central Committee of the Association in the United States, and enter into regular correspondence with the National Committee. ... It matters little whether you are followed by the Italians or not. It matters greatly that the National Committee should know with whom to correspond, and be able to simplify the work by concentrating it. The anti-papal work would pass into your hands. It may be very useful, but only on condition that Americans realize that the two questions—the political and the religious—cannot be separated, and that we, by overthrowing the temporal power of the Papacy, will destroy it spiritually as well. Books and weapons have the same value. The national revolution, by founding a Rome of the People, will put an end to the Rome of the Popes (*44* : 64–65).

The first task was to raise funds, and for that Mazzini conceived the grandiose plan to float in Italy and abroad a national loan of ten million francs, which was to be repaid with interest by the government of free Italy after the successful conclusion of the revolution. Mazzini hoped that a considerable sum could be raised in the United States. Italians there, he thought, would buy bonds out of patriotism, and sympathetic Americans would buy bonds as a tangible proof of their sympathy. Perhaps some American investor might be tempted to speculate by the offer of a large discount and the hope of realizing large profits in a short time. Mazzini believed that by organizing large mass meetings some of the political enthusiasm of the audiences could be converted in cash for the bonds, and advised Foresti along that line. Foresti, on the other hand, insisted that it was preferable to concentrate their efforts in the antipapal circles. Mazzini did not put too much reliance on the success of this scheme, because of his experience with the Christian Alliance.

I do not agree completely ... with your idea of not launching the Loan with great publicity by means of meetings. I am not acquainted with the United States, but they belong to the English race, and I know their customs. I am convinced that the moral advantage of a powerful echo of sympathy, coming to Italy from beyond the Atlantic, would be as great as the material advantage, and, if possible, should not be neglected. The meetings would be useful in two ways: to spread the sympathy for the cause, and to increase the number of subscriptions. The resolutions proposed should have, as a practical corollary, one stating that it is the sense of the meeting that the Italian cause should be aided by supporting the Loan. The bonds being offered on the spot, at the end of the meeting, they could be easily placed.... A few Americans were in Rome during the siege, and became enthusiasts. If one could be found to speak as an eye witness, it would be fine. I remember a young man, Strong, with his wife, Irish I believe. ... Mr. and Mrs. Spring, friends of poor Miss Fuller and mine, would help. ... Another person who could and would help you a great deal, is Miss Cushman, the actress. I know her, and I am writing to her, but it is necessary to send to her our acts, circulars, etc. Do not fail to do it (*45* : 59–61).

But in spite of all his urging and entreating, Foresti did not do anything, partly because he was old—over sixty by then—and partly perhaps because he was beginning to drift away from Mazzini, attracted by the monarchical idea which five years later won him over completely. And Mazzini a few months later complained that in all the United States they had sold one single bond and received only one single contribution of 250 dollars, which Mazzini received directly from Marcus Spring.

Hopes for the success of the loan in America were revived at the time of Kossuth's tour. After the fall of the Hungarian revolution, Louis Kossuth, accompanied by a few followers, had taken refuge in Turkey, where he was relegated to Kutaiah, a town in Asia Minor. Here Kossuth was the object of persistent demands on the part of Austria and Russia for his surrender and of England and America for his liberation. When Mazzini organized his European Democracy, he sent, together with the French, German, and Polish representative, an invitation to Kossuth to join in their work.[1] Expecting the revolution to take place within a short time, the participation of Kossuth was of great importance, not only because his personal popularity in England and America assured the movement a favorable press in those countries but also because the prestige of his name among the Hungarians could lead many Hungarian soldiers in the Austrian army to desert and join the rebels.

Kossuth, however, fully conscious of his political stature, was unwilling to allow the use of his name lightly. He doubted the wisdom of striking too close a relationship with men like Ledru-Rollin and Ruge who did not have too great an influence in their respective countries or Mazzini whose statesmanship he was inclined to doubt. Anticipating a Russo-Turkish war, with Austria siding with Russia, and England and France with Turkey, he expected the next Hungarian rebellion to be sponsored by the Western allies, and he felt he had to consider carefully the connection he made, lest his leadership be rejected as too radical by the governments of France and England when that time came. Thus when, after a silence of several months, he replied to Mazzini's invitation, he declined, because he could not afford, he said, to appear a "professional revolutionist"; but he promised to investigate the situation in Italy and confer on the possibility of a common action with him in London after his liberation.[2]

The coöperation of Kossuth was too important to Mazzini to let matters stand. Early in 1851, he sent to Turkey his friend Adriano Lemmi. Before 1848, this young Tuscan patriot had resided for many years in the Levant and had conducted there a prosperous importing business, in the course of which he had made numerous connections in the business and bureaucratic circles which he expected to use in his political mission. His task was to aid the American and British agents who were in Turkey to arrange and finance the flight of Kossuth in case diplomatic means failed to obtain his liberation. It was Lemmi who served as intermediary between Kossuth and Homes, the American agent there,[3] and who later arranged for Homes to consult with Mazzini in London (45 : 244, 299).

Meanwhile Kossuth, perhaps on Lemmi's suggestion but certainly with Lemmi's help, sent his faithful English friend, Captain Henningsen, to investigate the situation in Italy and ascertain the importance and strength of Mazzini's party. Aided by friends to whom Lemmi recommended him, Henningsen was able to visit the Neapolitan Kingdom, Tuscany, the Roman States, and Piedmont. He interviewed republicans and monarchists, extremists and moderates, conspirators and members of parliament, and at the end went to London to interview Mazzini himself. From there he sent Kossuth a long report[4] in which he described Mazzini's organization, "the efficiency of the invisible government [of the Mazzinians], the success of the National Loan, the high morale and the sentiment of discipline reigning among Mazzini's followers ... and concluded that this organization was very strong, was spread over all Italy, and that there was nothing to be hoped from the constitutionalists, nor from the royal house [of Savoy], but everything was to be hoped from Mazzini."[5] On the basis of this report, Kossuth accepted the proffered alliance and agreed to serve on the Central European Committee, more to please Mazzini, one is inclined to suspect, than because of real faith in its effectiveness, since he paid no attention to its other members and seldom even mentioned their names.

When at length Kossuth was liberated, before departing for the United States he stopped for a few weeks at London, where he was the object of enthusiastic popular demonstrations. Between rounds of public appearances he had a number of conferences with Mazzini, in the course of which they perfected their program of common action and cleared up some controversial points. Against the advice of many English friends Kossuth made an open confession of republican faith and acknowledged publicly his alliance with Mazzini. But he refused to agree to a complete fusion of the causes of the two countries, as Mazzini suggested. A few months earlier Mazzini had organized a Society of the Friends of Italy, to which belonged many eminent literary and artistic personalities— Walter Savage Landor, Professor Newman, David Masson, and Macready, among others. Mazzini now wished to change it into a Society of the Friends of Italy and Hungary, but Kossuth declined to concur. Having been the idol of his country during the revolution, the object of diplomatic action during his detention, and of enthusiastic popular demonstration after his liberation, both in England and America, Kossuth had not tasted yet, as he did later, the salty bread of exile, so often seasoned with the gall of disappointment, on which Mazzini had steadily fed for almost twenty years, and was inclined to look superciliously on that humble spade work of organization of favorable public opinion.

One of the plans discussed at that time was the invasion of Sicily, a plan first thought of before the return of Garibaldi from South America in 1848. The plan was much like the one successfully carried out nine years later in which one thousand soldiers landed in Sicily to start and direct the revolution there. Even before Kossuth left for New York, Mazzini wrote twice to Garibaldi, who was somewhere in Central or South America, to urge him to accept the command of the expedition (47 : 87–88, 116). Later, Adriano Lemmi, who accompanied Kossuth in America as his secretary, went to Malta to await there the shipment of arms the Hungarian was to purchase in America to outfit the expedition.

On December 4, 1851, Kossuth arrived in New York. He spent seven months in the United States, and his stay was a triumphant progress through the country, as far west as Saint Louis and as far south as New Orleans. He was received everywhere with wild demonstrations of enthusiasm. The ovation he received in New York by cheering crowds of hundreds of thousands of people was such that "the greatest of Roman generals might have been proud of such a triumph," as an American historian put it. "It was, indeed, a curious spectacle," commented the same historian, "to see the descendants of sober-blooded Englishmen and phlegmatic Dutchmen roused to such a pitch of enthusiasm over a man . . . whose only title to fame was that he had fought bravely and acted wisely in an unsuccessful revolution."[6]

Mazzini, who by that time was well aware of the touch of egotism in the character of his Hungarian colleague, had written to his friends in New York hinting that they would do well to keep their enthusiasm within bounds. "Italian welcome to Kossuth," he advised, "but with dignity, speaking as one nation to another, as one power to another, so that he feel the need of maintaining a loyal alliance with us" (47 : 91). But it must have been difficult to remain cool in the midst of the universal enthusiasm. Failing to obtain a prominent place in the official parade, the European Democratic Committee organized a parade of its own two days after the official reception, in which there were almost seven thousand persons, two German bands and one Italian band, and a display of the red flag of democracy and the national flags of Italy, France, and Poland. Arriving at the Irving House where the Kossuth party was staying, General Avezzana presented the red flag to the Hungarian patriot, who accepted with the expressed reservation that he was not a socialist.[7] "In my opinion," he said in reply to Avezzana's address, "Democracy is a principle, and Socialism is a system. My unreserved adhesion is for the former. . . . It is not for me to inquire nor to judge what system may best suit the political and social wants of other countries; but as far as my own is concerned . . . I am convinced that Hungary does not want nor wish for the application of any system of socialism. I may add, on the authority of statements made to me by Mazzini, that Italy, too, in this respect is quite in the same predicament."[8]

Kossuth's object was to rouse public opinion in England and America to such a crusading pitch against European despotism that it would determine their governments' attitude on a policy of aid and comfort to the European revolutionary parties. In America his propaganda turned on two main themes: one was that the United States, in opposition to the interventionism of the Holy Alliance, should proclaim the doctrine of self-determination of peoples the basic law in international relations and assert its readiness to enforce such a law; the other was a restatement of the American policy of recognition of all *de-facto* governments enjoying popular support, irrespective of their legitimacy, and insistence on the right to trade with such governments in peace *and war*. The advocacy of such a militant policy ran counter to the traditional policy of neutrality of the United States, as Kossuth well knew and as he was emphatically reminded by Henry Clay in an interview the American statesman had with the Hungarian patriot. But Kossuth argued that the policy counseled by Washington to the infant struggling republic of 1796, whose only duty was "to grow, to grow, and still to grow," was no longer suited for the young giant of 1851. The United States, standing powerfully over a whole continent, needed to fear no country on earth and had to assume the duties of leadership the newly acquired power was forcing on them.[9]

It was not only out of a sense of duty that America had to accept its position of leadership in the world but also out of enlightened self-interest, of self-preservation pure and simple. The coalition of despotic powers could not allow the prosperous progress of a free country which, by its mere existence, exerted a subversive influence over the oppressed people of the despots. The despots had to destroy the free countries so that they themselves might continue to live. "While the tree of freedom which the Pilgrims planted," Kossuth told an audience at Plymouth, Massachusetts, "grew so high that a twig of it may revive a world, in Europe, by a strange contradiction, another tree has grown in the same time—the tree of evil and despotism. It is Russia. Both have grown so large that there is no more place for them both on earth. One must be lopped, that the other may still spread."[10]

A few days later Kossuth took up this point again in Salem, Massachusetts. In that address he gave an analysis of the irrepressible antagonism between the United States and Russia which is worth re-reading for its astonishing present-time flavor one hundred years after it was first presented.

All sophistry is in vain, gentlemen; there is no mistake about it. Russian absolutism and Anglo-Saxon constitutionalism are not rival but antagonist powers. They cannot long continue to subsist together. Antagonists cannot hold equal positions; every additional strength of the one is a comparative weakening of the other. One or the other must yield. One or the other must perish or become dependent on the other's will. ... Gentlemen, I have often heard the remark that if the United States do not care for the policy of the world, they will continue to grow internally and will soon become the mightiest realm on Earth, a Republic of a hundred million energetic freemen, strong enough to defy all the rest of the world, and to control the destinies of mankind. And surely this is your glorious lot; but only under the condition that no hostile combination, before you have in peace and tranquillity grown so strong, arrests by craft and violence your giant course; and this again is possible only under the condition that Europe becomes free and the league of the despots become not sufficiently powerful to check the peaceful development of your strength. But Russia too, the embodiment of the principle of despotism, is working hard for the development of her power. Whilst you grow internally, her able diplomacy has spread its nets all over the continent of Europe.

The despots are all leagued against the freedom of the nations; and should the principle of absolutism consolidate its power, and lastingly keep down the nations, then it must, even by the instinct of self-preservation, try to check the further development of your Republic. In vain they would have spilt the blood of millions, in vain they would have doomed themselves to eternal curses, if they allowed the United States to become the ruling power on earth. ... How could they permit you to become so mighty, as not to be not only dangerous by your example, but, by your power, a certain ruin to despotism? They will, they must, do everything to check your glorious progress. Be sure, as soon as they have crushed the spirit of freedom in Europe, as soon as they command all the forces of the continent, they will marshal them against you. Of course they will not lead their fleets and armies at once across the Ocean. They will first damage your prosperity by crippling your commerce. They will exclude America from the markets of Europe, not only because they fear the republican propagandism of your commerce, but also because Russia requires those markets for her own products. Russian diplomacy will foster domestic dissentions, and rouse the South against the North and the North against the South, the seacoast against the inland states, and the inland states against the seacoast, the Pacific interests against the Atlantic interests; and when discord paralyzes your forces, then comes at last the foreign intervention. ... And Europe being oppressed, you will have, single handed, to encounter the combined forces of the world.[11]

In many of his speeches Kossuth made frequent references to Italy and its revolutionary spirit which under the leadership of Mazzini was striving to win its freedom from domestic tyrants and foreign oppressors. "Fair, but unfortunate Italy, which, in so many respects, is dear to my heart," he declared at the dinner of the Press in New York. "We have a common enemy; so we are brothers in arms for freedom and independence. I know how Italy stands, and I dare confidently declare there is no hope for Italy but in that great republican party, at the head of which Mazzini stands. It has nothing to do with communistic schemes or the French doctrines of socialism. But it wills Italy independence, free and republican."[12] He repeated these expressions of sympathy and solidarity at Harrisburg, where he explained that Italy failed in 1848 because at that time "the spirit of Italy was divided between Charles Albert, Mazzini, and the Pope," but that now the Italians "know their aims, and are united in their aim, and are burning to show the world that the spirit of ancient Rome is resurged in them."[13]

The second speech at Faneuil Hall on May 12, 1852, was almost completely devoted to Italy, "the sunny garden of Europe, whose blossoms are blighted by the icy north wind from St. Petersburgh," "the captured nightingale, placed under a fragrant bush of roses beneath an ever-blue sky!" Kossuth defended the courage and military skill of the Italians questioned by the supporters of absolutism by recalling that many great military leaders of the past—Piccolomini, Montecuccoli, Farnese, Eugene of Savoy, Spinola, Bonaparte—were Italians. Only the power of Austria kept the Italians in fetters, and Austria was able to hold its sway because of the Russian support, without which it would be power-less. "No revolution in Italy was ever yet crushed by their own domestic tyrants without foreign aid." "Remember that one-third of the Austrian army which occupies Italy, are Hungarians, who have fought against and triumphed over the yellow-black flag of Austria under the same tricolor which, having the same color for both countries, shows emblematically that Hungary and Italy are but two wings of the same army, united against the same enemy." In Italy the spirit was ready and the organization was perfect. And here drawing liberally and even quoting literally from Hen-ningsen's report, Kossuth described with picturesque details and amusing anecdotes, the organization in Rome of the secret govern-ment of the revolutionists whose orders were obeyed by the popu-lation and feared by the minions of the petty tyrants.[14]

Kossuth did not hesitate to bring up the points on which he disagreed with his Italian ally, at times needlessly so. At the con-gressional banquet in Washington, he advocated a federal union for Italy, though he must have known that Mazzini had been opposing such a plan with all his strength since the beginning of his political activity.[15] At Columbus, Ohio, he referred deprecat-ingly and condescendingly to the eagerness and impatience of Mazzini: "Circumstances will grow over my head, and men may take the destinies of nations into their hands, who, perhaps, even as faithful as I—as, for instance, Mazzini, with whom I am on very friendly terms, but who is, perhaps, not as skilled in the school of practical misfortunes as I am—will spoil it all."[16]

The splendid reception accorded to him by the people and government of the United States, the words of sympathy and encouragement he heard from leading political figures, and the definite promises received from glib politicians raised Kossuth's hopes to a high pitch at the very beginning of his American tour. On December 22, 1851, from New York he wrote jubilantly to Mazzini as follows:

Here things go superlatively well—better than I had hoped. The policy of indifference to European affairs will be completely changed into an active policy favorable to us. The American fleet in the Mediterranean will be re-inforced to protect their trade with us, in spite of all the pro-tests of our enemies; any revolutionary government will be recognized at the very beginning of its existence, and will be able to grant letters of marque, and to buy anything it wants here, freely and openly. I will also have money; you can count on my buying, in a few months, five hundred thousand francs of your bonds—in ready cash. ... You cannot imagine the change I have been able to cause in the political opinion here. Every other question is pushed into the background, foreign relations dominates everything.[17]

This letter was brought to Mazzini by his friend Lemmi, who had accompanied Kossuth to America as his secretary and had returned to Europe to go to Malta and wait there for a shipment of arms for the Sicilian expedition. Undoubtedly Lemmi reported verbally on the enthusiastic welcome Kossuth had received in New York, which must have filled Mazzini with high hope for the success of Kossuth's mission and his own national loan. He replied immediately: "I have seen Lemmi and received your letter of December 22nd. God bless you for your efforts and for the laborious task you have undertaken for the good cause" (*Appendix, 6 :* 160). Upon Kossuth's promise to buy, within a short time, half a million francs worth of Italian bonds, he hastened to send the bonds to Foresti (*47 :* 161), taking the occasion to spur his friend to greater activity for their sale among the Italians. "When Americans give for Hungary," he wrote, "Italians should give for Italy. Of the bonds of the Loan, I think you have sold only one. Considering the fact that many Italians live in the United States, it is almost incredible. Think about it, and try to urge them, wherever they are, to make this act of patriotic faith" (*47 :* 163).

It is difficult to get a clear picture of the relations between Mazzini and Kossuth during the latter's tour of America, because, as usual, only part of their correspondence is extant. For the seven months Kossuth spent in America we have ten letters Mazzini wrote to him and three that he wrote to Mazzini. There are references to at least three or four more not yet discovered. The correspondence available suggests that the plan on which they had agreed before Kossuth's departure was based on a repetition of the events of 1848, when the revolution in France gave the signal and the stimulus to movements in the rest of Europe. Their task now, waiting for that signal again, was to perfect the secret organization in Hungary and Italy; to organize the military forces available among the exiles for an expedition that was to serve as the rallying point of the revolution; to propagandize Italian troops in Hungary and Hungarian troops in Italy to refuse to fight the rebels and perhaps even join them; to organize sympathizers abroad, especially in England and America, in order to obtain financial help during the preparations and diplomatic support after the revolution; and, finally, to build stores of arms and ammunitions for the initial blow.

Louis Napoleon's coup d'état of December 2 upset these plans and spread discouragement in the camp of the revolutionists. Mazzini hastened to reassure Kossuth that disappointing as the new turn of events was it left the situation unchanged in Italy and Hungary and that France itself was not lost to the cause, because the opposition to the "pretender" was very strong and would be felt as soon as the exceptional military regime was lifted, as it had to be sooner or later, because, "you can support yourself on bayonnets, but you cannot sit on them" (*Appendix*, 4: 153–55). He even saw a silver lining in the concern of England over the "plaster replica" of Napoleon his nephew was trying to cast, which concern made English public opinion more sympathetic to the national movements (*Appendix*, 4 : 155–56, 166; 47 : 155). But he had finally to admit that paralysis had seized the Hungarians in London and that the work of preparation agreed upon was at a standstill.

One way to offset the loss of France, Mazzini thought, was to work out an understanding with the Spanish republicans for a synchronization of a Spanish revolt with the Italian revolution which would put Louis Napoleon between two fires. The Spanish republicans were well organized but disarmed, because their government had been buying up their weapons. Could Kossuth arrange to have the Americans supply them with seven or eight thousand rifles? In exchange the Spaniards were willing to cede all their presidios on the African coast except Ceuta.

In addition, in return for real support in arms and money [Mazzini wrote], the Party would be willing to cede Cuba, which would mean American domination of the Gulf of Mexico. Besides this material aid, they would like the United States to give moral support for a reunion of Spain and Portugal. This union, which would remove Portugal from the all powerful British influence, is the desire of the Spanish National Party, and is widely accepted by the influential men of the Party in Portugal. Meanwhile, if you can make some propositions to the United States, and if these propositions find a favorable response, an American delegate should come to Europe. I would put him in direct contact

with the leaders of the movement, and they could come to an understanding. These chiefs are in France and Spain (*47* : 239–40).

Kossuth was skeptical about the possibilities of Spanish coöperation. He found Mazzini's reasoning about the rearming the
Spanish republicans rather peculiar, since it amounted to rearming
people who had sold their own weapons.

You tell me [he replied] that Catalonia and Aragon could rise tomorrow
if they did not lack arms. And you add, "the government has taken care
of it by buying up their rifles." But, good heavens, can you believe
seriously that men who sell their arms to the government for a few
miserable colons are on the point of revolting? I have taken the steps
you suggested in this connection, dear friend, being careful not to say
a word about this sale of arms. Nevertheless this is the answer I received:
"You realize that there is nothing to be done with the government
of the United States. You know the statement to Congress concerning
Cuba by the Fillmore administration: that is sufficient to show that
this administration will never enter into relation with the Spanish
republican party before it becomes government." So it was only the
"Cuban" party that I could approach. This I did. The Spanish republicans had anticipated you there. Before coming to you, very cleverly,
they had begun by sketching the future republican organization, in
which the abolition of slavery was established. That is fair enough, but
if one makes such a decision, he should not approach America, where
the "Cuban" party and the political flirtations with Cuba, are based on
the speculation of having an extra weight for slavery, to counterbalance
the weight of California and Oregon. In short: they reject with indignation any advance of this kind from the Spanish republican party.[18]

After Kossuth promised in his first letter from New York the purchase of a large amount of bonds of the Italian loan, Mazzini frequently reminded him of that promise. No need, Mazzini suggested,
to wait until the entire half a million francs could be purchased.
"As soon as you have a fraction available, you should send it," he
wrote on January 13, 1852 (*47* : 156). A few days later he mailed a
package of bonds to Foresti and reminded Kossuth: "Remember
that Foresti has a deposit of our bonds, and you only have to ask
him for them. If you succeed in getting some funds for this
purpose, send them on gradually" (*Appendix*, *4* : 164). On April 19,
he reminded Kossuth once again: "You have not said a thing
further about the Italian Loan" (*Appendix*, *4* : 171); and five days
later he wrote: "If you have some money, remember your promise
for the Loan" (*Appendix*, *4* : 172). But time went on, and Kossuth

never sent any money. As a matter of fact, when he returned to London he was not able for some time to repay a loan of five hundred pounds Mazzini had had a group of his English friends raise for his voyage to America. In his last letter from New York, Kossuth explained why no funds were available and gave a list of his expenditures, showing that in December alone he had used over sixty thousand dollars for rifles, rounds of ammunition, and propaganda. And Mazzini sadly informed Lemmi, still waiting in Malta: "Substantially, from the last letter Kossuth wrote to me I gather: that he has no money at all; he spent whatever he collected and made some additional commitments. He will not give you money; he will not give me any either. About the bonds, not even a word; ditto, about the five hundred pounds of the Englishmen. He ruined me instead of helping me. Morally he did much good, more perhaps than he himself realizes now, but the result will not be apparent until after the start of the revolution" (47 : 299).

This partially negative estimate of Kossuth's tour was what the Hungarian himself had given in his last letter.

I am leaving America, where, with much effort, I have accomplished a great deal for the future, but almost nothing for the present. For the future the result is: that once the revolution starts, the Americans will rush to aid us in every way. I say "us" because I never spoke of Hungary without speaking equally of Italy, as of an identical cause, and without making clear that whatever they do for Italy will be done for Hungary as well. Also, whatever the new administration may do in the United States, it will have to take an active part in European affairs. Every revolutionary government will be recognized immediately; the Mediterranean Fleet has already been strengthened, the old admiral replaced by another, the order forbidding American officers to speak of politics rescinded; the fleet will protect the American trade with the revolutionary governments.[19]

Mazzini explained Kossuth's failure to his friends who had been led to expect great immediate results by pointing out that as Louis Napoleon's coup d'état had discouraged Italians from contributing to *their own* cause so it had naturally lessened the interest of foreigners who were asked to give for someone else's cause (47 : 317). Contributions amounting to more than forty thousand dollars had been withdrawn in the United States as soon as the situation looked less promising for an immediate revolution. "The fact is that the moral result obtained in America is im-

mense: we shall have large means, and help both official and non-
official. But no one will help those who do not do anything, and to
expect others to make our revolution is madness" (*47* : 342–43).
Mazzini continued to believe firmly in this future aid of America
through the period of Pierce administration. His own will to
believe was greatly strengthened by the grandiose promises of
Young America. The retirement of the leading members of Young
America from their official positions and the quiet dissolution of
the movement itself convinced him eventually that no help could
be expected from that quarter.

Chapter VII

MAZZINI AND YOUNG AMERICA

~~~~~~

"Young America" was the name taken by the radical wing of the Democratic party, which under that slogan attempted to win control of the party during the Presidential Campaign of 1852. The name was chosen by obvious analogy with the various "young" movements that flourished in Europe in the thirties and forties. The first to use the term in a political sense and to formulate a program of action was Edwin de Leon, who in a commencement address at South Carolina College in 1845 remarked that as there were a Young Italy, a Young Germany, a Young Ireland, there might as well be a Young America. "If there was to be a Young America, then the new generation, the young men of America, would have to express their faith in the glorious destiny of the country, by seizing political power to hasten the fulfillment of that destiny."[1]

What was an oratorical phrase in 1845 became a political program in 1852. The popular enthusiasm aroused by Kossuth indicated that the advocacy of militant liberalism might pay handsome political dividends. As the *New York Herald* put it, the cause of Hungary skilfully played might win the White House. Thus Young America came to the fore, with a program of economic and geographical expansion in the American continent and intervention in favor of the national movements in Europe.

The leader of the movement was George N. Sanders, who became editor of the *Democratic Review* in January, 1952. In his journal Sanders conducted a preconvention campaign attacking the "old fogies," the men in control of the party at the time, and demanding a new leadership more jealous of the country's honor and with keener perception of its real interest. The group was particularly strong in the Mississippi Valley and California, though some supporters were found in other sections of the country. Prominent among them was Pierre Soulé, U.S. Senator from Louisiana. Their favorite candidate for the Democratic nomination for president was Stephen A. Douglas. When Douglas failed to win the nomination, however, they rallied to the support of Pierce, hoping that he would develop into the type of leader they desired.

Sanders had close connection with Kossuth during the latter's tour of America, and remained in correspondence with him for many years after his return to Europe. He made grandiose promises of aid to the Hungarian. One of his promises envisaged the purchase, arming, and equipping of a fast American steamer, probably the one to be used for the Sicilian expedition. Other supporters of Pierce made even more fantastic propositions. William J. Stillman tells of one which assumed an astounding credulity on the part of the Hungarian patriot.

A presidential election was near and negotiations were initiated between Kossuth and the party leaders for his influence on the foreign vote. ... I was in the habit of going to see him at night, and sometimes waited for the departure of the committees of politicians who were in discussion with him. One night, when I went in, I found him in a state of nauseated irritation, and he broke out, saying, "Mr. Stillman, if your country does not get rid of these politicians it will be ruined in fifty years!" He had just received a Democratic Committee, which had formally promised to him in return for the influence he might exert in favor of their candidate, two ships of war ready for service, and a sum of money, the exact amount of which I cannot remember, but I think it was half a million dollars. ... The Committee had presented itself with the authority of Franklin Pierce.[2]

First through Kossuth, then directly, Young America gave verbal aid and comfort to Mazzini also. That support, though limited to promises, came opportunely at a time when the fortunes of his party were at a low ebb because of the failure of the Milanese uprising of 1853. A number of workers' associations plotted a revolt in Lombardy. Of the several groups that were to rise simultaneously in various parts of the city, only one moved on February 6, 1853, the day appointed for the insurrection in Milan, and the affair ended in a short bloody affray and was followed by the violent reprisals of the Austrian authorities. Though he had no part in planning the uprising and had only consented to give whatever support he could to the movement, Mazzini accepted all the blame for the failure in order to shield some undiscovered leaders of the plot. As a result many of his followers deserted his flag—a blow from which the party never really recovered.

The promises of aid from America served as a badly needed tonic to the flagging faith of the remnants of the republican organization. Letters written by Mazzini to his lieutenants in various Italian centers—to Giacome Acerbi in Genoa, Ambrogio Ronchi and Massimiliano Grazia in Milan—are replete with detailed assurances of help from the United States as soon as the revolution should begin. In July, 1853, he wrote to Acerbi as follows:

We have won over two important elements on which the attention of our party must be called: at home, the Hungarian element, which has been tested in ten different localities, and found everywhere with us; abroad, the American element, from the time of Pierce's election. To you I can tell that Kossuth and I worked for his election on the German element, very numerous in the United States—on some conditions, which he accepted. Of these conditions he has now fulfilled enough to reassure us that he will fulfill the rest. He was to appoint American agents in Europe who would sympathize with and help us, and almost all his appointments have been as we desired them. He was to give instructions hostile to Austria and to the despotic governments, and he did so—as proven by the conduct of the captain of the frigate at Smyrna. He promised to instruct his diplomatic agents to recognize *immediately* any revolutionary republican government established in some province of Italy or Hungary—and he affirms he has done so. This would be something of vital importance, because then the help prepared by American societies could come to us, without any hindrance from the government; also because, once we were recognized, we could easily involve them more deeply; also because we could then grant letters of marque, and fill the Adriatic and Mediterranean with American consuls hostile to Austria; and because of numerous other reasons. It is understood that neither the Hungarians nor the Americans can start our revolution. We must act. Help will not fail to come (*49* : 279–80).

The following month he wrote to Ronchi in a similar vein.

You know the change of policy toward us obtained in America. We are in excellent relations with the President; we received promises of which the instructions given to their diplomatic agents—whose tenor is revealed by the Smyrna incident—are a clear indication. Soulé, ambassador of the United States at Madrid and close friend of the President, who came to see me a few days ago, has brought a comfirmation. If a revolutionary republican government is established anywhere in Italy, it will be immediately recognized. ... Once a government is recognized, the individual Americans will have the right to help it: the aid is ready, and it will bring about the war. Moreover, we will be able to grant letters of marque to sea captains who will prey on Austria. But all this is dependent on our action. The same applies to the Hungarian movement, and many other things. We cannot expect others *to start our* revolution (*49* : 316–18).

The same assurances are found also in manifestoes and circulars issued in 1853 and 1854. In the manifesto *Agl'Italiani* (To the Italians), he asserted that partly through the influence of Kossuth public opinion in England and America was turning favorable to the republicans and that America was gradually abandoning its traditional policy of isolation (*51* : 33, 51). In the *Circolare del Partito d'Azione* (Circular of the Action Party), he asserted that in foreign countries, especially in the United States, there was sympathy for their cause—a sympathy which would become active at the first sign of life (*51* : 165). In the *Proclama Insurrezionale* (Insurrectional Proclamation), he repeated that in America there was openly proclaimed sympathy and deposits of arms for the revolution (*51* : 251). In the *Istruzioni della Giunta Nazionale d'Azione* (Instruction of the National Action Committee), he pointed out that the United States had long desired the annexation of Cuba and that Pierce, fully realizing that the program of American expansion fitted in with the revolutionary plans of the republicans, would not want to miss the opportunity "to enrich with another star the flag of the American Union" (*51* : 319–20).

It was all wishful thinking, of course, but the words and actions of some American representatives abroad were such as to make it plausible, especially to the republicans who wanted to believe it. The Koszta affair, which Mazzini quoted to his friends, was a case in point. Martin Koszta, a Hungarian refugee compromised in the revolution of 1848, had resided in the United States for almost two years and had made a legal declaration of intention to become a citizen when he happened to visit Smyrna on business. The Austrian consul there first tried to have him extradited; when that failed he had him kidnapped by some Greek gangsters and carried aboard the Austrian brig-of-war *Huszar* at anchor in the harbor in spite of the protests of the American consul. The American sloopof-war *Saint Louis* arrived at Smyrna shortly afterwards, and its captain was appealed to for help. After repeated requests failed to obtain Koszta's release Captain Ingraham trained the guns of his ship on the *Huszar* and threatened to open fire unless the prisoner was set free. The Hungarian was released into the custody of the French consul, and the controversy was eventually solved diplomatically in the sense desired by America. The vigorous action of Captain Ingraham excited European republicans, especially when they learned that in answer to Austrian demands for his punishment he was given a vote of thanks in a joint resolution of Congress and a medal was conferred upon him.[3] It is small wonder that Mazzini took the Smyrna affair as a proof that instructions hostile to Austria had been given to the captains of American warships.

Several appointments of diplomatic and consular representatives were such as to justify Mazzini's qualification "favorable to us." Sanders at the consulate of London, Soulé at the embassy of Madrid, Daniel at the legation of Turin, A. Belmont at the legation at The Hague, T. S. Fay in Switzerland, and John L. O'Sullivan in Portugal, were all members or sympathizers of Young America. Even Foresti, the acknowledged leader of Young Italy in New York, received an appointment as Consul in Genoa, which the Sardinian government refused to accept at that time.

The arrival of Sanders in London in November, 1853, inflated the hopes of the republicans. His home at London became their headquarters. Through him Mazzini obtained American passports for himself and his friends with the greatest ease.[4] Aurelio Saffi, one of the Triumvirs of the Roman republic, was given an American passport under the name of William Thompson, with which he traveled and conspired freely in Switzerland (*52* : 16, 53) in spite of the fact that he had been expelled from that country the year before (*53* : 85–86). For Caronti, another friend, Mazzini obtained not one but two American passports (*52* : 164–65) and a promise of a new passport from the American minister in Turin (*52* : 168). To Crispi he sent a blank American passport, to be filled out by him with his name and description, which represented him as a naturalized citizen (*54* : 150).

There was a deliberate ostentation in Sanders relations with European republicans, as if he wished to flaunt his connections with "subversive characters" and shock and alarm both the "old fogies" at home and the despotic governments on the continent. On the occasion of Washington's Birthday in 1854, Sanders gave a party for the leaders of the European republicans. To make sure that it was truly representative, the list of guests was prepared in consultation with Kossuth and Mazzini. In a letter dated Saturday, February, 1854, Kossuth wrote to Mazzini as follows:

As for Worcell you are absolutely right. Thank you for the suggestion. Sanders doesn't ask for anything better than to follow our advice. As far as I know there will be besides you, Ledru-Rollin, Garibaldi, and myself—Buchanan (the Ambassador), his private Secretary Welsh, Sir Joshua Walmsley (who surprised me by accepting eagerly a dinner of such marked character), the American banker Peabody, I believe, probably Pulszky. That is all that I know. I will warn them about Richard. He insisted on inviting L. Blanc, in spite of his socialism. But I did not know what suited you and Ledru-Rollin, and for that reason I was not able to answer him. What do you think of it? In case he should not do, what would you think of Pascal Duprat or Félix Pyat?

As a matter of fact, "it is a great bore this dining." But these Americans are like that—like children. The purpose, however, is good. It is to establish and display openly some secret connections between American diplomacy and the European revolution—and to include even some conservative bankers like Peabody. Let them have their way. If there is no profit, there is no loss . . . .

In short, he and the other (with whom we argued a bit the other evening at Sanders') are doing and will do all that we can reasonably ask them (except to give money). This goes to the point that if the supreme moment comes, and we need to send the final word to Pesth, Milan, Rome, to hell itself, one of them will carry it, and will do all we ask—you can be sure of it.[5]

At that dinner was present also Felice Orsini, the friend and fellow revolutionist of Mazzini who a few years later was executed for his attempt on the life of Napoleon III. He related that, among others, there were present the American Ambassador, Sanders' wife and children, Garibaldi, Herzen, Ledru-Rollin, Mazzini, Kossuth, Pulszky, and Worcell. "It was a magnificent dinner. There were no political discussions. We spoke of travel and American things. All European papers spoke of the banquet, and each, according to its political inclination, built on it the strangest and most absurd fancies" (50 : 139). Aurelio Saffi, who was also present, related, however, that toasts were drunk to the future alliance of the United States of America with the United States of

Europe.[6] Buchanan jokingly asked Mrs. Sanders "if she were not afraid the combustible materials about her would explode and blow us up." But in a serious vein he explained to the Secretary of State his presence at such an assemblage which could not but appear significant. "However indiscreet," he wrote to Marcy, "it might be for me, as American minister to invite them to my house, I should feel myself degraded as an American citizen to have refused the invitation of a friend, simply because men who have suffered in the cause of liberty were to be present."[7]

That dinner must have caused considerable comment in America. Four years later when Sanders was Navy Agent in New York and was entertaining lavishly in his apartment at the National Hotel in Washington, the *New York Herald* referred to this and similar political dinners of his and called him "a political philosopher of the carnivorous tribe." "Let us cite," the paper said, "a few of these notable dinners of Sanders. His campaign of 1852 against the 'old fogies' was commenced with dining and wining caucuses in New York, and then, with the nomination of poor Pierce, our eating philosopher went eating his way among the democracy. Sent over as Consul to London, we next find Sanders involved in a red republican Continental revolution, inaugurated in the disguise of a dinner to the revolutionary refugees in London. Recalled, however, by the 'old fogies' of the Senate, this scheme of eating and drinking up the despots of Europe was cut short, we think, at the third dinner."[8]

But besides these significant dinners, which the exiles understood perfectly to be window dressing of some sort, Sanders promised them aid of a more substantial nature. A few years back he had bought from the War Department 144,000 obsolete rifles; he had sold some to Kussuth[9]—perhaps the 15,000 rifles Kossuth purchased in December, 1851, for $35,000[10]—but he still had a considerable number to dispose of, and the European republicans were the best prospective customers. These must have been the weapons which Mazzini in 1854 assured his friend that the Americans were holding in readiness to support European revolutions. In letters to Fabrizi (*52* : 174; *53* : 13) and Massimiliano Grazia (*52* : 318) Mazzini gave assurances that as soon as a revolt began he would be able to buy rifles—payment delayed—from American friends who had them stored in the Mediterranean area and at Constantinople.

Ironically enough, this line of propaganda on American aid later boomeranged on Mazzini when, for example, he asked his friends in Italy to raise twenty thousand francs and was told that he should try to get it from the Americans (*53* : 184) and when Pisacane demanded a share of "the huge sums recently received from the United States" for his ill-fated expedition to Southern Italy (*54* : 329). Needless to say, Mazzini had never received any "huge sums." He received scarcely any contributions at all except in promises—promises that galled him, especially when during the Crimean war he felt confident that, given the means, he could lead a successful revolution in Italy because the powers, distracted by the events in Turkey, would be unable to interfere.

I have been on the Continent till now, [he wrote to Foresti on December 24, 1854,] and I shall return there shortly. I cannot stay away from the frontier, in the hope of doing something. If we let this war end, we are cowards and unworthy of liberty. . . . What do your Americans say? Ah! if, instead of colossal promises for later, they understood that a little help given before would change the situation completely! If an association, a man, realized that the relatively small sum of fifty, thirty, twenty thousand dollars in my hand, would open a vast camp of sympathies, influence, progress, and glory for America! (*53* : 298).

Even after the Senate refused to confirm his nomination to the consulate of London, Sanders continued to wage his verbal war on European despots. On August 21, 1854, the London *Times* published a letter he addressed to the President of the Swiss Confederation protesting the abridgment of the right of asylum recently enacted by that country.[11] His feelings were echoed shortly thereafter by Theodore S. Fay (not Fey, as Mazzini wrote), the American Ambassador to Switzerland, obviously another sympathizer of Young America, when someone asked him what he would do if Mazzini were arrested in that country. "If Mazzini were arrested," he was reported to have replied, "I would immediately use all my influence with the Federal Council, and this in the name of my government, who certainly would not disavow me—to prevent that he be handed over to France, or Austria, or Piedmont. I would take him under my protection, and although he is not an American, it would be in the name of the Great American Republic, in the name of Humanity, in the name of all the popular sympathies that surround Mazzini that I would consider my duty to protect him" (*53* : 129–30).

All these activities, declarations, and gestures of American representatives caused some alarm and annoyance in the cabinets of the continental powers. Indeed, since the election of Pierce, to whose nomination Kossuth contributed with a circular to German societies and clubs in America, the French and the Austrians had shown some concern. The *Journal des Débats* and the *Revue des Deux Mondes* saw the election of Pierce as ominous for the peace of Europe.[12]

In contrast, Mossi, the Sardinian chargé d'affaires in America, did not seem much impressed by the possibility of an alliance between the American government and the European republicans. From 1850 on he reported faithfully to his government the activities of the Italian clubs in New York and the movements of Garibaldi while he was in America. When a committee was set up to organize in a "Patriotic Legion" the exiles who were ready to return to Italy for a war of independence and to raise funds for their passage home, he reported the names of the members of that committee, among whom were Foresti, Avezzana, Forbes, and Filopanti, to his government "so that the government could take measures for their expulsion from the Kingdom should they succeed in entering it." But he expressed assurance that the "committee was not dangerous or to be feared." As to the possibility of an Anglo-American rapprochement for a common action in support of liberty on the European continent, Mossi sagaciously commented as follows:

As to the probability that this government allow itself to be drawn into an active role in European affairs, the thing is altogether absurd, and does not deserve any attention. Even supposing that the incoming administration is democratic, and that they decide to modify the policy of non-intervention followed until now by the United States, it will nevertheless be very difficult for them to act in accord with Great Britain against Russia and Austria. The hate and wrath of the Democratic Party against Great Britain are too strong and deep, to make possible the rapprochement necessary for a sincere common action.[13]

The same skepticism was expressed later by the Sardinian press about the rumors of large shipments of American arms to the republicans. Commenting on these rumors the Turin *Opinione* of April 28, 1854, stated:

The correspondence of some English papers from New York informs us that 200,000 rifles were loaded in that city for a mysterious destination. It is assured that 100,000 have been assigned to France, the others to be distributed among Ireland, Hungary, and Italy, in proportion to the needs of the revolution. These guns supposedly have been bought in London with Russian money, and put at the disposal of Mazzini and Kossuth, and, in order to assure, besides the Russian aid, also the active support of American democracy, the plan has been made to inveigle the United States of America in a war against France and England, to which the pretext would be given by the island of Cuba, whose possession was guaranteed to Spain by these two powers. The plan is not badly conceived, and the alliance between Mazzini and Nicholas is at least original. For the present, however, there are still a few little obstacles to its execution. President Pierce of the United States is inspired by peaceful ideas toward Spain, and does not wish to engage in a war to satisfy the desire of European demagogues, and the *Black Warrior* affair which was to be the spark, has already been composed in a friendly way; the immense majority of the population of the United States is opposed to Russia as much as all Western Europe, and would not want to start a war with France and England for the advantage of Russia, for the simple motive that, while the commercial relations with the former countries have an immense extent, those with Russia are hardly perceptible. ... A slight doubt arises that the 200,000 rifles, like the above mentioned projects, exist in imagination, rather than on the ships sailing from New York (*52* : 126–27).

Italian diplomats devoted much more attention to, and showed more concern over, Pierre Soulé when he was appointed Ambassador to Madrid. Mossi informed his government of the political antecedents of Soulé and ventured the opinion that "one should not be surprised if the Cabinet of Madrid decides not to receive him." Just before Soulé's departure from America, Mossi reported, he was given an ovation by the Cuban refugees. "This ovation was quite imposing: the Cuban refugees were joined by several members of the extreme democratic party who, longing for the annexation of Cuba, have formed an association named the *Lone Star*, whose goal is to prepare the means to take the island from the Crown of Spain."[14]

In August, 1853, on his way to his residence in Madrid, Soulé stopped at London, where he met with the republican exiles (*49* : 317) and brought to them decisions made by Young America which Kossuth had been expecting for months. Perhaps it was he who brought confirmation of the offer of warships and guns—an offer withdrawn a few months later because of an antislavery letter of Mazzini, according to the complaint of Kossuth. "America is lost," Kossuth wrote to his Italian friend in December, 1853. "The offer of warships and of 35,000 rifles has been withdrawn; three of my financial committees have dissolved—all because of your letter. The administration uses it as a pretext to say, 'We cannot do anything for you because Mazzini roused the jealousy of the Southerners; we cannot do without their support, therefore we must withdraw from you!' Two years of work lost! It is irreparable!"[15]

When in October, 1854, Soulé met with Mason and Buchanan at Ostend to discuss ways and means to induce Spain to part with Cuba, the European diplomatic circles buzzed with rumors about the purpose of the conference. Since the Ostend Manifesto was not published until several months after the meeting, rumors persisted for a long time that its purpose was the organization of insurrections in Europe—a suspicion made plausible by the fact that after the Ostend meeting Soulé went to London and conferred with the republican exiles there. Marquis Antonini, Ambassador of the King of Naples in Paris, reported in October to his government:

A rumor goes around here, with assurance of certainty, that this imperial government has had in its hands the threads of a republican conspiracy intimately connected with the demagogic activities of Spain. It is also said that the notorious Mr. Soulé, envoy of the United States at Madrid, is one of the most enthusiastic supporters of the propaganda of the *Universal Republic*, and that he has been the most acrimonious instigator of the democratic insurrection which has taken place in his residence. Moreover, it is said that a conference was held among several envoys of the American Union to work out together a plan of general insurrection in Europe. It is further said that Mr. Soulé, after having taken part in this conference, and after having held several meetings with the leaders of the revolutionary emigration, was not allowed, by order of this imperial government, to cross France to return to his residence in Madrid.[16]

Soulé felt confident, as he wrote to Marcy from London on October 20, that in case of war with Spain, France and England would not be in a position to interfere because of their commitments in Crimea.[17] But it is possible that as a sort of insurance he planned on stirring some republican trouble on the continent in case war with Spain should come. He informed the republican leaders in

London that he had funds from some mysterious source to aid them.

Mazzini was on the Continent at the time Soulé visited London. When, on his return, Kossuth gave him a report on his conference with Soulé, he saw a chance to secure the funds he needed for the Italian movement, and immediately cast about for a safe way to have a letter delivered personally to the American diplomat (53 : 300). Dall'Ongaro in Brussels found someone who expected to go to Madrid on some personal business, but was not able to go to London for an interview. Consequently, Mazzini explained the situation in a letter.

Soulé has in deposit a sum destined to European things. The problem is to get a part of it. I would write to him, but a letter of this kind is not sent by mail; besides, the bearer should add a few words to persuade him. If the person of whom you speak accepted, the trip could be made immediately, and it would not be necessary for him to come and see me beforehand. I would send the letter for Soulé, and from the letter itself, from some notes I would prepare, from a conversation with you, and from his own convictions, he would get what he would need for the hortatory part of the conversation (53 : 341).

While waiting for completion of the arrangements, Mazzini heard the news of Soulé's resignation, which made a special trip to Madrid useless (54 : 18). Still, knowing that the fund held by Soulé was not connected with his official position, he decided to write and send the letter to Dall'Ongaro to forward to America.

I am sending the letter to Soulé [he wrote], one for Perceval, and a little note for Orense. Read them all and comment upon them. . . . To Soulé I ask *less* than I should, if he is inclined to give. To you I say that I would be happy if I had, within a week, ten thousand francs. I am spending my own money as much as I can, but as my ill fortune would have it, the little I possess is so tied up, that it will not be available for six or eight months. Some expressions in my letter to Soulé allude to an idea I have as to the source of the fund that I know for a fact he has. I know he alluded to it with Kossuth when he asked for me in London during my absence (54 : 100–101).

In his letter Mazzini expressed the opinion that the Republicans in Europe could not afford to let the end of the Crimean War come without taking some action. If they did, and peace was concluded, the result would be the domination of Europe by a new Holy Alliance, with Austria made the keystone of European despotism, the Napoleonic usurpation strengthened for at least ten more years, England tied to the status quo, and America excluded from all influence in Europe for many years. Italians realized that the time to act had come. They had been waiting, up to that time, for an offer of support by either side of the belligerent powers, but they knew now that they had to rely on themselves. Would Soulé care to help?

So that the movement may be strong and be in a way the spark that set fire to the train of powder, I need some financial help. I have some means, but it is not sufficient. Complete it! I could, if necessary, try to complete it elsewhere, but in that case I would have to reveal my secret, and very probably some imprudence might make it public. I know— some of your countrymen and Louis Kossuth affirm it—that some funds are in your hands destined to the support of the cause of the nationalities, and to extend the influence of the United States on the path of the Good; you can at once attain this double aim. Put in my hands a part of this fund. Fifty thousand francs would put me in condition to overcome many difficulties; one hundred thousand francs would put me in a position to face them without hesitation, and successfully (*Appendix, 5 : 52–53*).

As a guarantee Mazzini offered his entire life devoted to a single aim, the considerable influence he enjoyed with his countrymen, and some experience. America could count on the gratitude of the Italian people, who would aid with all their power the influence of the United States in Europe. As for the chances of success, Mazzini felt he could guarantee the success of the revolution; as for the war that would follow, he could not be equally certain, but even for that he had reasonable hopes of success, because a sizable part of the Austrian forces were occupied elsewhere, and because the Italian revolution would be the signal for other revolutions in Europe.

There is a reference to the mysterious source of the fund allegedly held by Soulé. Was it Russia? Mazzini felt he could accept the aid, irrespective of the source.

From whatever source this fund comes, I feel I can accept it. I cannot betray my principles, and I do not have to discuss anything but the domestic question. It is the Sovereignty of the Country which our movement will invoke: the nation will judge what suits them best. But to any man in power I wish to say, "I am an enemy of Austria; I intend to attack her, and I feel strong enough, with some help, to pin down her forces in a domestic struggle. If there are some who believe that this operation may be useful to them, and wish to contribute to its realization, they will be my strategic allies: politically I have no alliance except with my country" (*Appendix*, 5 : 54).

Though sent to Dall'Ongaro, this letter never reached Soulé. With the resignation of Soulé and the recall of Sanders, whatever influence Young America may have had with the administration disappeared, and the group itself quietly dissolved. The appointment of Breckenridge of Kentucky, one of the "old fogies," as Soulé's successor to Madrid underlined the fact that the republicans could not look to Washington for support of their schemes. Mazzini had no further contact with Soulé. He was in correspondence with Sanders as late as the end of 1858.[18] Since most of Sanders' letters are still unpublished, it is impossible to say of what importance they are. It is not likely, however, that they may reveal any new schemes, since the influence of both Sanders and Mazzini had declined too far to allow them to make any plan with even an illusory chance of success.

Chapter VIII

THE LECTURE TOUR OF
JESSIE WHITE MARIO

Mazzini's popularity in America followed, naturally enough, the same trend it did in Italy: it was at its highest peak after the gallant defense of the Roman republic; it began to decline after the attempted revolution of Milan in 1853; it declined even further as the prestige of the Savoy monarchy rose following the Crimean War; and it reached its lowest level in the late fifties because of the Genoese revolt of 1857, Orsini's attempt on the life of Napoleon, in which Mazzini was at first believed implicated, and the war of liberation of 1859, which marked the definite acceptance of the monarchical leadership on the part of the Italian liberals.

In the early fifties America felt sympathetic and at times even enthusiastic toward Mazzini. Dailies such as the *Tribune*, the *Herald*, the *Times*, periodicals such as the *Democratic Review*, the *International Monthly Magazine*, the *Boston Weekly Museum*, were unanimous in their praise of the Italian leader and the political trend he represented. The Address of the British Society of the Friends of Italy to America, which Lemmi brought in 1851, was sympathetically received, though its appeal was not given the practical response that was hoped for. Mazzini was acclaimed for his "unsullied moral purity," his "utter abnegation of self," his courage. To the Catholics who accused him of extreme radicalism, of socialism, and even communism, it was replied that Mazzini had Washington as his model and that he was the "apostle of the doctrines on which American institutions rested."[1] It was affirmed that to him rather than to the House of Savoy the Italians should look for leadership in their struggle for freedom. Only the conservative *North American Review* expressed distrust, as early as 1849, for the work of secret societies and conspiracies and preference for a constitutional monarchy under the leadership of moderate liberals of the type of Balbo, Gioberti, and D'Azeglio.[2]

The Milanese revolt of February 6, 1853, was strongly criticized in the American press. Though Mazzini and Kossuth were still hailed as "the noblest champions of human rights in Continental politics," it was deplored that they allowed their hopes to mislead them into starting revolutions which were bound to fail because of the conditions of Europe. The Milanese revolt did prove that the temper of the Italians was such that foreign domination and Papal rule would soon be cleared out of the land; but it was doubted that the political future of the peninsula would be republican.

The Crimean War and the subsequent peace marked an important point in the history of Italian liberalism. The leadership of Italian liberals was definitely taken over by the Sardinian monarchy. Manin, the leader of the Venetian republic of 1848, accepted the program of a united Italy under the constitutional monarchy of the House of Savoy, and many, indeed most, republicans followed him. One by one most of Mazzini's friends and followers sacrificed their personal preference for a republic to the monarchical plan, which offered a greater chance of success. Indeed, Mazzini himself was willing to yield to the monarchical leadership, provided the monarchists would agree to submit the constitutional question to a constituent assembly as soon as all Italy was free.

As the monarchical faction gained ground in Italy so it did abroad. The American press became increasingly more sympathetic toward the House of Savoy. It was pointed out that the House of Savoy had a well trained army that had shown its mettle in the Crimean War and had the diplomatic support of France and England, its allies in that war. The Republican party could count on no foreign sympathies and support and militarily had to rely on untrained levies which, as shown by the campaigns of 1848, were no match in the field for regular armies. Many exiles accepted the Savoy monarchy—among them Foresti, who for so many years had been the loyal, if not able, lieutenant of Mazzini in the United States. "My soul is bitter," wrote Mazzini to Foresti on February 10, 1856. "With our best in prison, with almost all the men of 1848 and 1849 led astray by dreams which are at times shameful, we

have started on the very road of systematic inertia which lost for
Poland all European sympathy, and almost the right to exist"
(*56* : 112). A few months later Foresti, too, was lured by the
"shameful dream" of political regeneration through the monarchy,
and returned to Italy as American consul at Genoa.

The attempted revolution in Genoa in the Spring of 1857 elicited even stronger criticism, and the attempt by Orsini on Louis
Napoleon's life provoked outright indignation. The purpose of
the Genoese revolt was not to attack the Sardinian monarchy but
only to secure arms for the Pisacane expedition against the Kingdom of Naples, the ill-fated forerunner of the brilliant and successful filibustering expedition led two years later by Garibaldi. The
American press criticized Mazzini sharply, and even the *Tribune*, so
partial to the Italian leader, could find only an extenuation in the
fact that the exiles, brooding over a single idea, had become
monomaniacs and had felt justified in adopting the same principle
followed by their enemies, namely, that the end justifies the means.
After the attempt on Louis Napoleon's life, many papers which
a few years earlier had paid homage to the virtue and devotion
of Mazzini referred to him as that "wretch."[3]

There is no indication in Mazzini's writings that he was concerned or even aware of this change in American public opinion
toward him. However, some of his friends were, and one of them,
Jessie White, a young English writer who had just completed a
successful speaking tour through England and Scotland in
behalf of the Italian cause, suggested to him early in 1857 the
plan of a lecture tour in America. Mazzini approved of the idea
and even discussed some details connected with it, such as the
offer of naval stations to America in exchange for American help
(*58* : 34), but occupied as he was then with the preparations
for the Pisacane expedition, he suggested that a serious consideration of the project be postponed. "I do rather believe in the success of the American scheme," he wrote to her in March, 1857,
"but it is now either too late or too early; and you know why.
There would be no practical result for what I am trying. If that
vanished or failed, then the scheme might be resorted to. Summari-
ly, the little good that can be done, must be done quick and near.
Within two months you shall be free to reject altogether or to
discuss the American proposal" (*58* : 50–51).

The scheme was held in abeyance for almost a year. First Jessie became involved politically in the Genoese revolt of 1857 and was arrested and imprisoned for several months by the Sardinian authorities; then she became involved romantically with the Italian patriot Alberto Mario whom she later married in England. It was not until the following year that the plan was discussed again. This time it was expanded to include a role for her husband, Alberto Mario, who was to try to awaken the Italians in America while Jessie appealed to the Americans (*60* : 378).

Early in the Summer of 1858 the preparations for the trip began in earnest. Both Mazzini and Kossuth wrote to America to find sponsors for the lecture tour (*61* : 64) and to make preparations for the organization of a committee there to take care of all practical arrangements (*61* : 66, 91, 116). Letters of introduction for the Marios, besides Mazzini's and Kossuth's, were obtained from English friends, among whom were Mary Howitt and J. D. Morrell;[4] and the financial arrangements were completed. The trip was financed to a large extent from funds supplied by Mazzini. Alberto Mario wanted to consider Mazzini's 120 pounds sterling as a personal loan, but Mazzini insisted that they were going on a mission and that the expenses were to be paid by the party. If and when they felt prosperous they could if they wished make a gift to the treasury of the party (*61* : 194–96).

On October 26, the Marios sailed for the United States. Since clouds of war between Austria and France over the Italian question were gattering on the horizon and the feelings of the Italian people were running high, Mazzini thought that it was desirable to have his program presented once again to the American people in order to win public opinion and support in case the situation should offer him an opportunity to seize control of the movement. "The probability of a crisis of war for the coming year," he wrote to Alberto Mario, "is growing ever more. Let's then strengthen ourselves, gather means, and close the ranks of the party, so as to be able to govern ourselves according to circumstances with a certain degree of power, in addition to that of the Truth, which is on our side" (*61* : 372).

The task of Alberto Mario was to reorganize the Republican party among the Italians in America. For this purpose Mazzini prepared for him a careful and detailed set of instructions for organizing the party in the various cities. Among them were the following points:

You must try to organize the Party among the Italians in all points you will visit in the United States.

In New York you will see Avezzana and Ancarani about the popular element. You will insist on the necessity of a practical organization of the Party, on the formation in New York of a Central Section for the United States of America; on the formation, hence, of a Committee for the Section. You will ask for introductions for Boston, where is a certain Bachi, a Sicilian, once very active, later fallen asleep: wake him up. [Bachi had passed away five years before.] From him and from New York you will get addresses for Philadelphia, New Orleans, etc.

It seems to me that when you arrive at a place you should request authoritatively the Italians with whom you come in contact, to call together on a certain day in some large room, all the Italians reputed good, to give them a communication from the National Action Party. Recommend that they include the working people, who are always more ready to welcome proposals of activity. Once gathered, speak to them as a Representative of the Action Center; tell them that the Party is being reorganized everywhere; tell them of the duties of the Italians residing abroad; tell them that those duties are imposed upon them not only by their country, but also by European public opinion; tell them that this revival of the Party is universal, from South America to the seaports of the Orient; tell them about the duties that are laid on us by our martyrs, our Nicoteras in prison, etc.; tell them all that God and Country inspire you to say. Then proceed to the two forms of organization and activity: propaganda, and preparation for action. Explain our organization, the monthly contributions, the Fund for the Action, etc. Request them to form a Section of the Party *ipso facto*, and to set up a Committee of three to direct the two special committees— Finance and Organization. Request them to obtain a number of subscriptions for the paper, and to supply us with the address of a bookseller or someone else, that we can publish in the paper. Take down the address of the Committee, and pass it on to us; give them my address and that of the Finance Committee here. It is better that every State correspond with us, unless you are certain that the Committee in New York is as active as the undertaking requires. And give me, as you go on, a few lines of report. In short, what Mrs. Mario will do with the Americans you will do with the Italians. Although on a relatively smaller scale, the results may be very important for us. . . . To you I need not say anything else. If there is a chance of success, you will succeed (*61* : 299–301).

During their six months' stay in the United States, the Marios corresponded fairly regularly with Mazzini. Unfortunately the Mario letters are not extant, and the sad story of the tour must be pieced together from Mazzini's letters and from reports in the American press. The tour started rather inauspiciously. Arriving in New York early in November, they were condemned to one month of inaction because the people they had been recommended to were still away from New York and because the necessary preparations had not been made (*63* : 22, 25, 29–30). But eventually the arrangements were completed, and Jessie began her series of lectures under the sponsorship of a group of eighteen leading citizens of New York, among whom were prominent politicians such as Hiram Barney and George N. Sanders, the eminent barristers David Dudley Field and William Maxwell Evarts, the well-known clergymen Henry Martyn Field, George B. Cheever, Henry Whitney Bellows, and Henry Ward Beecher, and the editors of the *Times* and the *Tribune*, Horace Greely and Henry J. Raymond.[5] Indeed, the list of sponsors read like a Who's Who of New York intelligentsia in the late fifties.

The lectures were delivered at Clinton Hall in Astor Place from December 1 through January 5. The general topic was "The Religious, Social, and Political Aspects of the Italian Question." From newspaper reports we gather the following lecture schedule: December 1: "Italy and the Papacy"; December 8: "The first martyrs of Italian liberty"; December 15: "The revolution of 1848"; December 20: "The heroic defense of Venice and Rome"; and January 5: "The future plans of the Republicans."

The thesis that Madame Mario presented to her audience was that the fundamental obstacle to Italian liberty was the military power of Austria. The native rulers of Italy were in reality puppets in the hands of Austria, and had neither the power nor the willingness to take the leadership in the fight for the liberation of the country. The burden of the first three lectures was that Italians could not look for their liberation to their native princes, because both remote and recent history gave abundant proof that the Popes, the King of Naples, and the King of Sardinia never had the interest of their country at heart.

The Papacy, she said in her first lecture, had always opposed Italian nationality, and had from the beginning always called in foreign powers to prevent the political unification of the peninsula —from Stephen II, who called the Franks against the Lombards in the eighth century, to Pius IX, who called the Catholic powers to put down the Roman republic in 1849. The amnesty granted by Pius IX on his elevation to the pontifical throne which had aroused so much enthusiasm had really consisted in emptying the prisons of the victims of Pope Gregory in order to fill them again with his own. "Such has been the condition of Italy under the papal rule that her martyrs now go to their death for their love of country, without any notice being taken of their fate. So frequent have executions become that men begin to regard them as ordinary occurrences. One would think that the steps of the scaffold were lined with velvet, so little noise do these young heads make in their fall."[6]

In her second lecture Madame Mario sketched the rise of the national spirit in Italy after the French Revolution and analyzed the repressive role played by the two Italian monarchies, Naples and Sardinia. The faithless Bourbons in Naples had shamelessly broken their pledge to their people in 1799 when they murdered the leaders of the Partenopean republic and again in 1821 when they persecuted the leaders of the Carbonari revolution. Charles Albert of Sardinia, "the traitor of 1821, the executioner of 1833," was likewise stigmatized for his relentless persecution of the patriots, among them Mazzini who was exiled because of a letter he addressed to the king on his ascent to the throne urging him to treat the Italians better than his predecessors had done.[7]

The third lecture told the story of the revolution of 1848, which, in the lecturer's opinion, had given rise to much misunderstanding in America. Many people shared the erroneous notion "that it was only kings and popes who acted well in 1848." The truth was that the princes had misunderstood, mistrusted, and misled their people to such an extent that a popular movement which should have achieved the independence of Italy ended instead in defeat. Official documents and diplomatic correspondence, she claimed, made abundantly clear that Charles Albert did not engage in the war against Austria for the independence of Italy but solely to aggrandize his dominions with the addition of some Lombard territory. He did not trust the people, and refused the help of volunteers. "Charles Albert did not use the people in his army because, he said, he did not want an army of enemies at his rear. The people were prevented from coöperating in the movement. The victories of the Piedmontese army took place when four republicans were at her head, and when they left, the reverses came."[8] "The lecturer argued," a reporter wrote, "that every social or political revolution on the Italian peninsula is due only to the people, and not to their kingly leaders. She maintained, by diplomatic correspondence copied from the *Blue Book* of England—the pages of which have been only accessible since 1854—that Charles Albert, the Sardinian king, though styled the defender of liberty, was a traitor to the Italians, and only engaged in the Lombard war in the hope of increasing his territory."[9]

The fourth lecture related the gallant defense of the two strongholds of the Italian republicanism, Venice and Rome, which fought stubbornly against hopeless odds to save at least the honor of the revolution when its fortunes were already lost. The flight of the Pope and his refusal to return to the capital as a constitutional monarch brought about the proclamation of the Roman republic, whose government elicited the admiration even of fair-minded opponents such as the British consul at Rome who spoke admiringly of the manner in which the Roman republic was run although he disapproved on principle of the republican form of government. Besieged by four foreign armies, Rome decided to make a stand, and "for two months the people stood up in Rome fighting for religious liberty and free institutions—and Protestant England and Protestant America stood by and saw the murder. Four thousand of Rome's sons lay dead upon the ground, and the French army entered Rome." Disclaiming any intention of giving an apology for the assassination, the lecturer referred to the recent attempt on Napoleon's life and asked whether Louis Napoleon, who had killed Rome, was not a greater assassin than Felice Orsini, who had attempted to kill Louis Napoleon.[10]

No detailed report of the fifth and last lecture has been located. The *Times* published only a short note on January 6, 1859, which read: "Signora Mario lectured last evening at the Clinton Hall to quite a small audience. Her statements with reference to the future plans of the revolutionists, though necessarily indefinite, were listened to with great interest." The *Tribune*, on the same date, published an even shorter note stating simply: "Signora Mario gave the last of her lectures on Italy last evening." It was evident that the interest of the audience had flagged considerably.

It was quite a come down from the first lecture which had been attended by a large and distinguished audience, according to the local press. The *New York Herald* reported as follows: "The fine lecture room at the Clinton Hall was very fashionably and largely attended, and there are few popular lectures so fortunate as to secure so large, intelligent, and appreciative audience on occasion of an introductory lecture. . . . The lecture began at half past seven o'clock, at which hour the hall was very comfortably filled, and visitors continually arrived in the course of the evening, so that up to nine o'clock, when the proceedings were brought to a close, there were some persons who had not heard anything beyond the concluding portion of the lecture."[11] The speaker and her topic were flatteringly introduced by Horace Greely, and the lecture was interrupted by frequent cheers and applauses. At the end, "a resolution was . . . passed, asking Signora Mario to continue her lectures, and the large assembly soon after separated, highly delighted with the amiable lady—several ladies and gentlemen taking the opportunity to be introduced to her."[12] Also, the *Tribune* reported that there was "liberal applause throughout, but the sentiment most prevailing, among the many ladies and gentlemen, appeared too deep to manifest itself in loud demonstration. Thanks were voted to the eloquent lecturer, and the course of lectures on the same subject was strongly recommended."[13]

Even allowing for the set phraseology of the reporters, it did seem an encouraging beginning. But Jessie must have felt some doubts about the success of the enterprise. She had come hoping to arouse interest in, and collect funds for, the cause of the Italian republicans, and she was finding it difficult even to make expenses with the fees of her weekly lectures. She must have written to Mazzini on the subject, because the latter wrote to a common friend: "No news from Jessie: I feel uneasy about her second lecture: it will be the decisive one. If she should lose by it, she will be compelled to give it up, and I shall have a real remorse. She will be ruined by debts . . . and partially so through me" (*63* : 49–50).

The second lecture, on which Mazzini pinned his hopes, was also attended by a large audience,[14] but instead of settling it stirred matters up by provoking a controversy between Jessie Mario and the *New York Times*. Commenting on Madame Mario's second lecture, which sharply criticized the Sardinian monarchy, the editorial writer of the *Times*, Dec. 13, 1858, after expressing full sympathy for the Italian cause and for the patriots who were giving their all for it confessed to a sense of weariness with all their agitation and propaganda that failed to be concretized in action. "As year after year this agitation passes by, as lecture follows lecture, and speech speech, and dinner dinner, we look for some tangible proposition, or plan of campaign, or scheme of general *soulèvement*, or something, in short, which history or experience, or common sense, fortifies us in believing will make an impression on a well organized and well officered army of two or three hundred thousand men." Mazzini's good speeches, able manifestoes, and noble thoughts were fine things indeed, but they did not achieve the independence of Italy. The time for stirring the national consciousness was past, because the popular mind in Italy was thoroughly stirred, and the readiness of the Italians to fight and die gallantly for their country had been abundantly proved by the revolution of 1848–49. But the experience of that period proved also that all that was not enough to win independence. They also needed "some plan of organization which should make their resistence in the field tenacious" and that would unite "the patriots of the various states in hearty cooperation." This plan and this rallying point, the *Times* felt, could be given to the Italian patriots by the Sardinian monarchy which Mazzini and his followers opposed so violently.

Madame Mario had denounced public opinion for scorning high-minded Mazzini as a failure and for singing the praise of scheming, treacherous Louis Napoleon, who "had been successful by wading through blood to the throne." The *Times* reminded her that the world can judge not the intentions but the results. "It judges of people's moral character by their lives and judges of their talents by the result of their labors. It concludes Louis Napoleon is a clever man because he has performed an exploit which requires a display of some of the highest moral and intellectual qualities. It concludes Mazzini does not possess executive abilities because he has never accomplished anything he set about. But it acknowledges . . . that while the former is a very bad man, the latter is honest and conscientious, and we think all this is perfectly reasonable."[15]

Madame Mario's reply, published in the *New York Times*, December 15, 1858, pointed out the inconsistency of judging people solely on the basis of success. Louis Napoleon, the great man of December 2, was the man considered a fool after his attempts of Strassbourg and Boulogne. If Mazzini had not yet achieved his goal of political regeneration of Italy it was because the obstacles met with in Italy, were greater and more numerous than those faced by any other country that ever had to free itself from foreign domination. It was not true that the republicans had no plan.

Mazzini has spent his life in teaching the Italians that since the Pope and foreign armies cannot be prayed or bought out of Italy, they must be fought out; that a popular insurrection is their only chance of success; that, until they cease to trust in princes and foreigners,—in anything, in short, save their own right arm—they will remain, and deserve to remain, a nation of slaves. . . . Their faith is sealed with the blood of their martyrs. From 1849 till the present hour, Italy has no exiles save the republicans. Her prisons are crowded with republicans, and the executioner's ax is sharpened for republicans alone. The flag of Savoy can boast of no martyrs because that flag does not represent a principle, but merely an expedient and a dynastic interest.

To the remark that Mazzini's work consisted in speeches, manifestoes and noble thoughts, she replied: "Mazzini's work now consists in organizing secretly Italian patriots within and without the peninsula, and from time to time a band of republican heroes appears on the battle fields to initiate afresh the revolution, and band will follow band, and the Italians will fight and fall, until the whole nation resound to the appeal."

The eventful years of 1848 and 1849 did not prove that the House of Savoy offered the best rallying point. "You say, 'Sardinia made the best and most promising resistance to Austria, that the Lombard army vanished before Haynau and Radetzki.' I reply that every inch of ground won by the Italians for Italy in 1848 and '49 was won by the republicans, and that at the close of that year Italy would have been freed from the foreigner, would have been free, independent and united, had not the monarchy stepped in and substituted the petty longings of dynastic ambition to the great national aim." In proof of this Madame Mario recalled that except for the fortresses, the popular insurrection had already cleared Lombardy and Venetia of Austrians when Charles Albert entered the fight to prevent, as he himself admitted, the proclamation of a republic in Lombardy. His appearance brought about disunity in the people; his insistence on immediate union of Lombardy to Piedmont resulted in the withdrawal of the other Italian princes from the war of independence; and when later the Austrians returned with reinforcements, he who had disbanded the people's army failed or betrayed the Lombards and concluded an armistice which surrendered Lombardy and Venice to the old masters. The following year when the fight was resumed "80,000 Piedmontese, with the exception of a few regiments, fled ignominiously before 60,000 Austrians, and the farce of Novara sealed the fate of Italy. It was left for republican Venice and republican Rome to wipe off the stain of cowardice from the Italian name—left there by royal treachery and royal flight—and they fulfilled their task."[16]

In his answer the writer of the *Times* declined to engage in a controversy on the campaign of 1849. He expressed surprise that Madame Mario would accuse 80,000 Piedmontese of cowardice, forgetting that Piedmontese, too, were Italians. The writer found natural that the King of Sardinia, believing as any king would that monarchy is the best government for a country, should want the annexation of the neighbouring states to his own. Certainly he could not be expected to abdicate and proclaim the republic, "dazzled no doubt by the brilliant success of other European republics." And he concluded by reminding Madame Mario that cookery books in giving the recipe for cooking a hare advised, as the first step, catching the hare.

For the manufacture of an Italian Republic, Italy itself is a prime requisite, and by the last account that country was held by 200,000 Austrian soldiers. . . . So we beg to advise the expulsion of foreigners as the first step, by any means and with any aid. . . . Submit to anything which shall rid the soil of the foreign soldiers . . . and place the government and destinies of Italy in Italian hands. When this is done, we shall be delighted to hear any observation which Mazzini may have to offer on the subject of the comparative advantage of a monarchy or republic.[17]

Madame Mario was taken to task for the charge of cowardice flung at the Piedmontese army by an anonymous Italian also who in a letter to the *Times* (December 17) suggested that her branding as cowards those who did not agree with Mazzini was doing more harm than good to the Italian cause and that certainly she did not represent the viewpoint of the majority of the Italians. A reply to the anonymous Italian was given by Alberto Mario in a short, belligerent note and by a number of Italians, led by Avezzana who wrote a long declaration affirming that the view of Madame Mario were shared by the majority of Italians. Avezzana stated that most

Italians were republicans and were opposed to the King of Sardinia and he confirmed Madame Mario's assertion of the ignominious flight of the Piedmontese army in 1849 and laid the blame and the shame exclusively on the leaders.[18]

The same argument was advanced by Madame Mario in her reply to the *Times*. It was a fact that the Piedmontese fled before the enemy in 1849, and it was also a fact that the Piedmontese were well known for their bravery. The contradiction was explained by the role played in the affair by the ruling class—the aristocracy, bureaucracy, etc.—of Sardinia which had consistently opposed the unification of Italy. This ruling class, or "monarchy" as Madame Mario termed it, realized that in a united Italy they would be swallowed up by the new ruling class that would arise in a united Kingdom of Italy, and for that reason they had hindered and would continue to hinder the unification of Italy, even against the personal desire of the king. It was they who had planned the defeat by sabotaging the reconstruction of the army, by inciting resentment against the Lombards, and by spreading defeatist rumors. That was the real reason why the republicans opposed the leadership of the monarchical faction; it was not merely their preference for a different form of government. If Sardinia were sincerely striving for the unification of the country, not merely scheming for some petty increase of her territory, no Italian, even of republican faith, would resist her leadership in the war of liberation, as the writer of the *Times* assumed.

If Sardinia, you exclaim, can send 80,000 men to the field for that purpose, so much the better; if she can supply stuff, *commissariat* and artillery, better still. And if she makes her own leadership in the movement a condition of her assistance, why, let her lead! If she asks to reign, let her reign! Ditto, cries every Italian I have ever known ... Mazzini ... from his first letter to Charles Albert in 1833, to his last pamphlet on the Genoese insurrection, has ever urged Piedmont to take up arms against Austria. Nor do I fear contradiction when I affirm that if Piedmont would declare war on Austria tomorrow, every Italian would follow her thankfully to the battlefield, and, in spite of their republican traditions and republican tendencies, would hail Victor Emmanuel King of Italy, even as they would have crowned Charles Albert in 1848. [19]

Another person who entered the controversy was Quirico Filopanti. A staunch republican, one of the leaders of the Roman republic in 1849 and together with Foresti and Avezzana an active member of the Mazzinian party in America in the early fifties, he had lately, like Foresti, accepted the leadership of the Sardinian monarchy for the sake of Italian unity and independence. From London he heard of the controversy between the *Times* and the Italian republicans, and sent an appeal to his republican brethren reasserting his constant faith in the republican creed but adding: "I am not so blind as not to see the impossibility of having an Italian Republic in 1859; and I am well aware of the fact that Italy, united under an Italian and constitutional King is preferable to Italy divided among many despots, both native and foreign." He concluded by urging his fellow republicans in America not to follow the suggestion of neutrality given by Mazzini if war should come between Piedmont and Austria but to aid in the fight for the liberation of the sacred soil of the country. "This result being once obtained, we shall put down our arms, and vote according to our opinion. If it be the opinion of the whole nation's majority, it will triumph; if not, it will be alike necessary and dutiful to respect their wishes."[20]

A separate but related controversy took place between Count Louis Kazinski, a Polish refugee, and Alberto Mario. In 1849, Count Kazinski along with many other Polish refugees had served in the Sardinian army which in that campaign had been under the command of another Pole, General Chrzanowski. He took issue with Madame Mario's criticism of Piedmont. He objected especially to her statements that Piedmont's liberal institutions were a sham and that Italian patriots who had taken refuge in Piedmont had been persecuted and many of them shipped to the United States. This last statement was a reference to the deportees on the Sardinian frigate *Des Geneys* whose landing had been the subject of controversy between the Mayor of New York and the Sardinian authorities four years earlier.[21] Kazinski recalled the tremendous sacrifices made by Piedmont in that campaign which, with the exception of a few Tuscan volunteers, she had to fight alone, and he justified the expulsions because the exiles had used "vile language and slanders against the present ruler and his government."[22]

The first reply to Count Kazinski's letter came from Theodore Dwight, Jr., who wrote a long and rambling letter relating the events he had witnessed himself in Turin in 1821 when Charles Albert as Prince Regent first accepted the leadership of the constitutional revolution, then recanted, fled the capital, and joined the enemy. The writer felt that Charles Albert had betrayed his country again in 1848; hence the Italian patriots were justified in denying confidence to any king and in depending only on themselves.[23]

More lengthy and detailed was the reply written by Alberto Mario, who gave a wealth of bibliographical references on the various charges made by his wife against Piedmont. The Italian people, Mario argued, owed no debt of gratitude to Piedmont for the financial sacrifices borne on account of the war of 1848–49, because the monarchy had undertaken those campaigns not for the independence of Italy but for the purpose of enlarging its territory. In other words, on their part it was merely a political speculation that went sour. For proofs he referred to the correspondence between the Minister of Foreign Affairs of Sardinia and the British ambassador in Turin and between the latter and Viscount Palmerston. To the monarchist assertion that only a few Tuscans aided Piedmont Mario replied that the Sardinian monarchy had deliberately rejected the aid of volunteers and of the Italian regiments deserting the Austrian army and that, in spite of that refusal, no less than 40,000 volunteers, besides the Tuscans, fought the Austrians in Lombardy and Venetia. As to the question of liberal institutions, he listed the repressive laws enacted in Piedmont during the last ten years; and, finally, in reply to the assertion that only a *few* political refugees had been expelled from Piedmont because of the vile language used against the government he gave a long list of eminent patriots who had suffered that fate and who could not be accused of unseemly language or conduct.[24] Count Kazinski replied two weeks later with a vague and inclusive letter which, with an editorial note, closed the controversy.[25]

In spite of opposition and criticism Madame Mario went on with her lectures. After completing the series in New York, she repeated it at the Athenaeum in Brooklyn,[26] and perhaps continued to lecture in New York on cultural subjects at Clinton Hall where on January 15, she delivered a lecture on "Illustrious Women of Italy."[27] On the previous day she had been the principal speaker at a mass meeting of European socialists. Here she gave an address on "The duties of the European people" in which each nation was assigned its specific task toward the common goal

of freedom from the "mongrel herd—kings, emperors, popes."
The task of the Germans was the destruction of the Austrian
Empire, "the rattlesnake, whose forked tongue envenoms all the
vital saps . . . the serpent who is at this moment stifling the life
breath of four valorous nations in its coils"; the task of the Poles
and the Italians was to destroy respectively the Czar and the Pope,
"the two centers of gravity of universal despotism." According
to madame Mario, the Catholic Pope represented "the Divine
Sanction of despotism over thought and conscience" and the
"Russian Pope . . . the brute force of despotism over the external
world." It is curious to note that General Avezzana who was to
give an Italian address at that meeting was not able to attend
because of "illness" and that none of Mazzini's friends was reported present. Evidently they were unwilling to be identified with
the "red republicans," with whom Mazzini differed unequivocally
and emphatically.

On January 17, the Marios went to Eagleswood, New Jersey, to
visit the school which Theodore Dwight Weld together with his
wife Angelina, the younger of the famous Grimké sisters, had
opened there a few years before for black and white children alike
with the financial support of Marcus and Rebecca Spring. She
addressed the pupils on the Italian question, and at the close a
collection amounting to $112 was taken to be remitted to Mazzini
for the benefit of his school in London.[28] Jessie must have struck a
friendship with the Welds, because she returned to Eagleswood
and visited there for some time in May after she had completed
her lecture tour. She spent her time there "working at something . . .
for the Press" (63 : 243), perhaps the *American Letters*, which she
published on her return to Europe.

In February, the Marios went to Washington, to the disappointment of the *Tribune* which regretted they had not been "deterred
by Kossuth's ill-reception among the slave holders and their
tools."[29] She delivered two lectures there on the fifteenth and the
nineteenth. At the second of her lectures one or two senators were
expected to speak in behalf of the Italian cause.[30] From Washington
the Marios went on to Baltimore where she delivered two more
lectures on March 10 and 21 at the Carroll Hall. The lectures were
announced in the local press in terms flattering to the lecturer.[31]
Possibly they went to New England later. From Baltimore Jessie
wrote to Mazzini asking him to write a sort of message or mani-

festo addressed to the people of New England. Mazzini declined to do so, feeling that it would sound "too dictatorial and bombastic" (*Appendix*, 6 : 19–20).

While Madame Mario went on lecturing in English, her husband addressed the Italian residents of the various cities they visited, trying to organize the Italian republicans according to Mazzini's instructions. Only one press report has been located of his speeches in the United States—the one delivered in New York on December 24, 1858, in Mr. MacMullen's lecture room at 21 East Twentieth Street. The lecture reviewed the elements of the war of 1848, the role of the Sardinian monarchy, and the prospects of the coming revolution which was anticipated within a short time. In accordance with the directions received from Mazzini, he presented the program and the organization of the Action party, and organized a section of the party at the end of the meeting.[32] He reported the outcome of the meeting to Mazzini who, although pleased with the result, expressed doubt that they would be able "to keep the corpse galvanized" after his departure (*Appendix*, 6 : 10). Later when Mazzini saw the text of the lecture he was greatly pleased with it, and he informed Jessie that long extracts from it would be published in *Pensiero e Azione* (*63* : 222). Alberto Mario held meetings of Italians also in Washington and Baltimore, at which meetings statements were signed supporting the stand Mazzini had taken concerning the imminent war. These statements were published later in the paper of the party (*Appendix*, *6* : 21).

From London, Mazzini followed with anxiety the fortunes of the Marios' tour. The month-long delay on their arrival caused him some concern, but he still hoped that when Sanders, Barney, and the others returned to New York they would display some activity. However, when Jessie was attacked in the *Times* and none of them came to her defense, he was disappointed. "You are a brave and noble woman," he wrote to Jessie, "and if you succeed, it will be all your merit. With Barney and all the set, I am thoroughly disgusted. If you only knew what prospects of activity he had offered to Kossuth and myself." (*63* : 101–2). As time went on, the financial condition of the Marios became embarrassing. Jessie wrote to some friend in England for a loan, and Mazzini, hearing about it, sent her 100 pounds with a gentle reproof: "I send 100 pounds," he wrote to her on March 4, "and, as I had offered, you

are wrong in not asking me. If more is wanted, we shall manage"
(*Appendix*, *6* : 18).

After the Baltimore lectures it was clear that the tour was a
complete financial fiasco. Jessie must have written to Mazzini
expressing her regret at having wasted precious funds and asking
his advice as to her next step. Mazzini answered with a delicate
and tender note on April 15, in which he said:

My deliberate opinion is that: 1, that you would be weak and not the
Jessie I know, should you make yourself miserable for one moment
about failure, money, and like things. It would imply an utter miscon-
ception of yourself, of me, of all those you love and who love you. You
have done your duty nobly and bravely; you have, owing partially to
me, tried an experiment, which it was well to try. If it is not as successful as we wish, the fault lies with the Americans, not with you. Morally,
you have done good; Mario has done good with the Italians. You both
have increased the chances of help, should we deserve it through action. As for money matters, you wrong at least me, if you torment yourself one minute about them. . . . You went for us; you have worked
for us; and why should you consider the unavoidable expense a loan, I
cannot imagine (*63* : 218–20).

By the time she received this letter, the war between the Franco-
Sardinian allies and Austria had begun. Jessie obtained some
contracts to cover the war for some American papers, and in July
returned to Italy. But no sooner had she set foot on the territory
occupied by the Sardinians than she and her husband were arrested. They were released later only through the intercession of
Garibaldi. On their release they were expelled, and had to sit out
the war in Switzerland until they were able to join Garibaldi's
expedition in Southern Italy.

CHAPTER IX

SLAVERY AND THE CIVIL WAR

MAZZINI always took a keen interest in the problem of slavery. As a school boy he read up on the slave trade and on the life of the slaves in America; as an old man, only two months before his death he wrote to a friend expressing a desire for some American correspondence, possibly from Garrison or some friend of his, on the condition of the emancipated slaves and other important questions (*91* : 343).

The paradox of the coexistence of slavery with free republican institutions cooled his enthusiasm for what he called "the ideal of liberty developing on the banks of the Potomac" (*6* : 106). To him, it constituted an embarrassingly telling argument in the hands of the opponents of the principle of popular sovereignty (*17* : 249) and a source of doubt to the believers of the republican faith. In his "Prayer to God for the Planters by an Exile," a short paper written for the Boston annual *Liberty Bell for 1846*, he called on the Lord to let the planters hear "the sorrowing cry of all who endure and fight for the Good in Europe, and whose confidence and faith is shaken by their stubborn crime;—the mocking cry of princes and kings of the earth, who, when their subjects are full of turmoil, point to the proud republicans of America, who alone of men maintain the helotism of pagan ages" (*29* : 291).

"To write one or two pages on abolitionism," he told the friend who requested him to write the "Prayer," "is just the same to me as to have to prove that the Sun gives light and warmth, or to prove an axiom" (*30* : 249). His opinions on slavery had truly an axiomatic character. Its existence denied the basic principle of the unity of the human race, the divine descendance of man, the law of progress by the unfolding of which man advances from slavery through serfdom and wage earning to final freedom. But these ideas were in him an intellectual conviction devoid of emotional surge. The problem of slavery was too far removed from his personal experience to stir him into an evangelical zeal for its abolition even remotely like his feelings for the abolition of "political slavery" of the white race on the European continent. Needless to say, of the social and economic problems with which slavery was connected in the Southern states he knew little and cared less.

He expressed admiration and sympathy for the work of the abolitionists in America (16 : 291), and counted John Brown among the martyrs for truth and justice together with Prometheus, Socrates, and Christ (76 : 34). When he introduced Marcus and Rebecca Spring to his friends in Italy, he always mentioned their activity in behalf of the Negroes as a title to special consideration. But this sympathy though sincere was not overwhelming, and one is tempted to doubt whether it could have borne the strain of a close association, since he was just as single-minded and exclusive in his idea as the abolitionists were in theirs. He was greatly annoyed by the effusions of the English abolitionists Th. Perronet Thompson and George Thompson, members of the Executive committee of the "People's International League" he had organized in England, because he feared that their "anti-American tirades" would hinder the organization of a similar association in America (33 : 105). He had no scruples about collaborating and conspiring with G. N. Sanders and Pierre Soulé, who were strongly opposed to the abolition of slavery. He tried to establish contacts between the Spanish republicans and American leaders interested in the annexation of Cuba, knowing well that this annexation was desired by the Pierce and Buchanan administrations for the additional political weight it would give to the slave-holding states.

These contacts with proslavery men alarmed at least one abolitionist friend of Mazzini, whom he reassured with the statement that they "never prevented me to express my conviction in favor of the holy cause of abolitionism" (53 : 342). And that was true. When asked to state his views on this matter, he always did so unequivocally. At the very time he was in close relation with Sanders and Soulé, he wrote two letters on the subject of slavery— one to Garrison[1] and the other to Dr. Beard of Manchester—

(*50* : 73; *52* : 222–23) which caused him some annoyances and arguments with Kossuth.

The letter addressed to the Rev. Dr. Beard, chairman of the antislavery committee of northern England, was in reply to an invitation to attend the committee's first meeting in Manchester. Mazzini apologized for his inability to attend because of poor health and pressure of other business, but he assured the committee of his complete sympathy with its aim and of his readiness to lend whatever aid he could for its success.

No man [he stated] ought ever inscribe on his flag the sacred word "Liberty," who is not prepared to shake hands cordially with those, whoever they are, who will attach their names to the constitution of your association. Liberty may be the godlike gift of all races, of all nations, of every being who bears on his brow the stamp of MAN, or sink to the level of a narrow and mean self-interest, unworthy of the tears of the good and the blood of the brave. I am yours because I believe in the unity of God; yours, because I believe in the unity of mankind; yours, because I believe in the educability of the whole human race, and in a heavenly law of indefinite progression for all; yours, because the fulfillment of this law implies the consciousness and the responsibility of the agent, and neither consciousness nor responsibility can exist in slavery; yours, because I have devoted my life to the emancipation of my own country, and I would feel unequal to this task, a mean rebel, not an apostle of truth and justice, had I not felt from my earliest years that the right and duty of revolting against lies and tyranny were grounded on a far higher sphere than that of the welfare of one single nation; that they must start from belief in a principle which will have sooner or later to be universally applied:—"*One God, one humanity, one law, one love from all for all.*" Blessed be your efforts, if they start from this high ground of a common faith; if you do not forget, whilst at work for the emancipation of the black race, the millions of white slaves, suffering, struggling, expiring in Italy, in Poland, in Hungary, throughout all Europe: if you always remember that free men only can achieve the work of freedom, and that Europe's appeal for the abolition of slavery in other lands will not weigh all-powerful before God and men, whilst Europe herself shall be desecrated by arbitrary, tyrannical power, by czars, emperors, and popes (*52* : 176–77).

The letter was published in the Manchester *Daily News* of May 30, 1854. Because of his well-known connection with European republicans, George Sanders felt called upon to try to forestall the impression in America that this letter represented an official view-

point of his friends on slavery. He wrote a letter to Kossuth—
Mazzini was absent from England—deprecating the agitation on
the slavery question in the United States and expressing the belief
that Mazzini's letter had no relation to it. Kossuth in his reply
agreed that Mazzini's letter was not related to the current agitation; he asserted that he personally, while deploring the existence
of slavery anywhere in accordance with his basic political principle, was against foreign interference in the domestic affairs of
another nation; and he concluded with the expression of a vague
hope that Americans would eventually abolish slavery by themselves, that "the American people . . . will of themselves, with all
the light before them, make their nation a model for every other."[2]

The equivocal stand taken by Kossuth succeeded in displeasing
everybody on either side of the question. It was naturally criticized
in the abolitionist press, both in England and America, and
compared enviously with Mazzini's forthright statement. F. W.
Cresson wrote in the *Anti-Slavery Advocate*: "It is a source of
much gratification that Mr. Mazzini possesses so much clearer
perception of human rights than does Mr. Kossuth; and that unlike the distinguished Hungarian, he will not allow the arts and
blandishments of republican slave-holders to cause him to swerve
one inch from the straight path of duty." The *National Anti-Slavery Standard* compared Mazzini, "that noble clear-sighted advocate
of Universal Liberty," with Kossuth, "a Man of Expediency, a
political trimmer," and concluded: "The letter is so noble in its
sentiments and presents such a marked contrast to the truckling
epistle of the Hungarian, that we cannot resist the temptation to
reproduce it. Behold the difference between the Man of Expediency and the Man of Principle." In a letter to the *Commonwealth*, a
group of German-American republicans asserted Kossuth was "a
diplomat and a politician, but not the man for rescuing the European Nations from the grasp of despotism" and called his letter,
"with its frosty and only theoretical denial of American slavery, . . .
a mean and cowardly act."[3] Disappointment over Kossuth's letter
was expressed also by Hawthorne, at that time consul at Liverpool,
to whom his London colleague had sent copies of his letter and
Kossuth's reply. "It was certainly pertinent in you," Hawthorne
answered, "to write the article which you now send me; indeed,
in the position which you hold in respect to Mazzini and his brethren, I think you are called upon to do it. . . . Now as to Kos-

suth's reply . . . I do not like it well enough to be glad he has written it. . . . Doubtless he says nothing but what is perfectly true, but yet it has not the effect of frank and outspoken truth."[4] As for Mazzini, he was completely disgusted with his Hungarian ally. "Yes, I have all that you sent about Kossuth and slavery," he wrote to Emilie Hawkes. "At the bottom of my heart I do not esteem that man; but he can still be useful. Besides, *alas*! my *great* Italians have deprived me of any right to be severe toward a Magyar" (*53* : 45–46).

Kossuth was annoyed with Mazzini and blamed him for his American woes, although he must have known that his unpopularity with the abolitionists was of long standing. During his American tour he had been constantly under attack by the abolitionists for his noncommital stand on slavery. Between December, 1851, and July, 1852—the time of his American visit—almost every issue of the *Liberator* carried some item critical of him, and often comparisons were made, even at that time, between him and Mazzini.[5] Garrison even made the muses contribute a long versified indictment published in the *Liberty Bell* for 1853 in which Kossuth, the false prophet of liberty, was apostrophized as follows:

> Far better for thyself, O Magyar Chief!
> And better for thy fallen country's sake,
> Hadst thou remained in exile, and constraint
> Of thine own freedom on the Turkish shore,
> Or perished in some Austrian dungeon drear.[6]

Mazzini again expressed his views on the question of slavery on the eve of the Civil War in a letter to Theodore Weld in which he reiterated his belief in the identity of the cause of the abolitionists in America with that of the European republicans.

We are fighting the same sacred battle for freedom and the emancipation of the oppressed—you, Sir, against *negro*, we against *white* slavery. The cause is truly identical; for, depend upon it, the day in which we shall succeed in binding to one freely accepted pact twenty-six millions of Italians, we shall give what we cannot now, an active support to the cause you pursue. We are both the servants of the God who says, "Before Me there is no Master, no Slave, no Man, no Woman, but only Human Nature, which must be everywhere responsible, therefore free." May God bless your efforts and ours! May the day soon arise in which the word *bondage* will disappear from our living languages, and only point out a historical record! And, meanwhile, let the knowledge that we, all combatants under the same flag, do, through time and space, commune in love and faith, strengthen one another against the unavoidable suffering which we must meet on the way.[7]

Mazzini was interested in the Negro Emancipation Society when it was organized in England, and inquired of Clementia Taylor about its immediate program and plans for the future (74 : 224). Later he joined it, declaring he was happy to take that opportunity to protest one of the "three things against which a man ought to protest before dying, if he wants to die in peace with his own conscience: slavery, capital punishment, and the actual either narrow or hypocritical condition of the religious question" (78 : 9). After the Emancipation Proclamation he stated that colored people should be granted full political franchise, because political liberty was the best guarantee of civil liberty, and because to deny them the right to vote would mean the re-establishment "in the republican lands of America, of the class of political serfs of the Middle Ages" (83 : 163–64).

His personal contacts with American abolitionists were few. Besides Marcus and Rebecca Spring, he was in contact with Gerrit Smith, Moncure Daniel Conway, William L. Garrison, and Sarah Remond. He met Conway, the Virginian abolitionist who was at that time minister of the Unitarian South Place Chapel in London, at Aubrey House, the mansion of Peter Alfred Taylor, M.P., an old and devoted friend of his. There he met also Sarah Remond, the sister of the eloquent colored orator Charles L. Remond and for a number of years the companion of Clementia, Mr. Taylor's wife.[8] He met Garrison in 1846 at the Ashursts', the English family that surrounded him with understanding and love and gave him a home in his exile.[9] Both Garrison and Conway spoke with admiration of Mazzini, and Mazzini expressed affection for Conway and the highest esteem and consideration for Garrison, although he differed sharply with them, especially with Conway, on some principles he considered basic in his creed—the principle of nationality and the use of force in a just cause. "There was a Mazzini cult," wrote Conway, "and to some extent my wife and I shared the enthusiasm, though we did not include in it any passionate interest in Italian unity. . . . Having lost my early devotion to the 'sacred soil' of Virginia . . . I could not share Mazzini's creed about sacredness of Rome and the importance of Italy's reintegration to the everlasting purpose." When on March 17, 1872, Conway held a memorial service for Mazzini in his South Place Chapel, he felt he "could say nothing about Italy. I could only speak of the fidelity and personal greatness of the man."[10] The one who was in closer agreement with him on the use of force, and perhaps on other points as well, was Gerrit Smith—the only one he never met personally.

During the Civil War, Mazzini's sympathies were naturally for the Union. In 1863 when Garibaldi took the initiative in Italy for a public expression of sympathy for Lincoln and the cause he was leading, Mazzini hastened to give his adhesion in an eloquent letter to the editor of the *Dovere* in which he said:

In these times of scepticism and moral inertia, when an invocation to a holy principle issues from powerful lips, every man has the duty to respond with firm voice, and express his faith in it. The principle in the name of which Garibaldi sends a salute to Lincoln—the principle that God has set as goal of the American battles . . . is the holiest possible. . . . It is the principle of Humanity. . . . It is the principle that states: God created not kings, masters and servants, but man, and cursed be he who violates its Unity, image of the Divine Unity. However the rays of the sun may color human features, wherever there is a heart open to love, and a face greeting Hope with a smile, and lips murmuring the name of God, there is a personality that no one can erase without crime, that must be allowed to bloom under the breath of fraternal love (*76* : 32–34).

But although his sympathies were unhesitatingly for the North, his reasons were not the same as those that determined the war between the states. Mazzini was interested in the abolition of slavery, but he was rather indifferent to the preservation of the Union. The American continent, he wrote to Clementia Taylor, was large enough for two or three confederations, though not large enough to allow a single inch of its soil to be polluted by slavery (*78* : 9–11). When, after the fall of Charleston, the issue of the Civil War had been decided, he repeated this view, and explained that he could not see how in a society based on individual rights, as he conceived America to be, a large section of the population could reasonably be denied the right to secede. If the decision were up to him, he would insist on the abolition of slavery and on an alliance against foreign threats, and then would allow the Southern states to keep their separate federation (80 : 126–27).

He was horrified by the assassination of Lincoln, and expressed concern over the effects it would have on the foreign and domestic policies of the United States. He foresaw that it would make the pacification between North and South more difficult, and feared that at the conclusion of hostilities America might turn against England rather than intervene in Mexico, as he understood Lincoln intended to do (*80* : 224–25). In March, 1865, he suggested to Karl Blind that he urge his friends in America to a crusade against the French in Mexico, "the enemy," and to oppose a war against England, which would be "useless, immoral, harmful," (*80* : 178). Later he expressed regret that at the time of the demobilization of its armies America had not encouraged its veterans to go to Mexico as "volunteers," because he felt that a common war against despotism would have helped to re-establish a fraternal feeling between the soldiers of the North and South (*81* : 276–77).

Mazzini and the other republican refugees in London had long regarded the situation in Mexico with anxious interest. In 1862, when England and Spain withdrew their forces from the Mexican expedition and it became evident that Louis Napoleon would continue his intervention alone, Mazzini, Karl Blind, and Ledru-Rollin decided to address to Lincoln an appeal for financial aid in order to stir up trouble for the French Empire in Europe. Their problem was how to send the appeal in order to be certain that it reached the President's hands. Mazzini knew personally two German liberals who were serving in the Union army, Major General Carl Schurz and Colonnel F. F. K. Hecker. He had met Schurz in London when the latter, though a mere youth of twenty-two, had already won quite a reputation in revolutionary circles for his part in the romantic rescue of Kinkel from the fortress of Spandau and had had a few interviews and some correspondence with him. Hecker he had met perhaps in Switzerland when the German leader had repaired there after the collapse of the Baden revolution he had led. Upon Mazzini's suggestion, the appeal was sent to Schurz with a request to pass it on to Hecker in case he felt he could not or would not deliver it to the President. Karl Blind wrote the appeal in which he asserted that the ulterior object of Napoleon's enterprise was the dismemberment of the Union and that the republican parties in Europe, in France especially, were eager to be of assistance to the American republic by assailing Napoleon in Europe. Garibaldi, who was later appraised of the plan by Blind during his visit in London in 1864, agreed to participate with an attack on the French garrison in Rome. Mazzini wrote the letter to Schurz in which the amount needed—five hundred thousand dollars—was specified (72 : 278–79). According to what Blind related, the appeal reached Lincoln through "a United States General," obviously Schurz, and "was received favorably. He reserved his final decision for the time of the crisis; but before that arrived, the hand of the assassin struck him down."[11]

Another incident somewhat connected with the Civil War in which Mazzini took great interest was the report of Garibaldi's possible acceptance of a command in the Union Army in 1861. After preliminary contacts lasting several months between Garibaldi and American representatives, on September 9, 1861, H. S. Sanford, Minister Resident of the United States at Brussels, went to Caprera, Garibaldi's island retreat, and in the name of his government offered him a post of Major General in the Union Army and the assurance of a large degree of freedom in the conduct of military operations. Garibaldi declined because he felt he could not be of help unless he had the supreme command of the Union army and unless he had also authority to abolish slavery in occupied territories. He, like Mazzini, made it clear that he was interested in the American war as a contest for the abolition of slavery, not as one for the preservation of the Union, which for Americans was still the avowed purpose of the conflict. For obvious constitutional and political reasons his terms could not be met, and no further discussion took place.

Although the negotiations between the American diplomats and Garibaldi were conducted with great secrecy, news of them began to leak out to the press on both sides of the Atlantic to the great consternation of the Italian liberals. Italian unification had been substantially achieved, but it was not quite complete. The events of 1859 and 1860 had gone beyond the most sanguine expectations of Italian liberals, and they now optimistically expected the momentum to continue and lead shortly to the liberation of the Venetian provinces from Austria and the freedom of Rome from Papal rule. For this crowning effort the presence of Garibaldi was necessary, both for his ability as a military leader and for his almost legendary personal prestige. In the absence of official news concerning the American affair the air was thick with rumors. On the very day Garibaldi had declined the American offer, a Turin newspaper published the news that Garibaldi had accepted the command of the American Federal Army. The Florence *La Nazione* stated what undoubtedly represented the feelings of all Italian liberals that "the arm of Garibaldi certainly could not serve a nobler cause, were it not that the supreme interest of his own country demand his presence here." Hundreds of petitions were circulated all over the country urging Garibaldi to remain in Italy and complete the unification of the country, with Rome and Venice as goals.[12]

Mazzini heard the news in London with shock and disbelief. On September 11, 1861, he wrote to Jessie White Mario:

> This very day, 11th, I read in the *Morning Star* that Garibaldi has accepted, under certain conditions, all American proposals! I do not believe in his going so far as to abandon his own country and throw discouragement everywhere. But if he does, I trust none of our best will follow him. Now more than ever, Venice claims us: there is the European initiative; and European liberty is the liberty of the whole world. . . . Whatever happens, I shall, as far as life allows, pursue my own work toward Venice, for the ensuing spring (*71 : 382–83*).

Four days later he wrote again to Jessie:

> If Garibaldi goes, he betrays his duty and his country shamefully. Those whom he invites to go, instead of obeying, ought to solemnly protest against his decision. We have Rome and Venice to emancipate; and by doing so, we would build a free anti-slavery Nation, and would be enabled to give far more powerful help to the abolitionists of America than by going and fighting their actual battles (*71 : 394*).

In order to keep "the General" home Garibaldi's followers rushed to organize some expedition either against the French or against the Austrians. Garibaldi wanted an attack on the Papal states. Mazzini preferred an invasion of the Venetian provinces. An attack on the French garrison in Rome, he thought, "would prove fatal," because they would have to stand alone against the Catholic powers, while in an attack on Austria they could expect the support of the other oppressed people of the Empire and thus "initiate the movement of European nationalities" (*72 : 39*). Garibaldi's views prevailed, and in 1862 the unfortunate episode of Aspromonte took place. Troops of the newly formed Italian army sent to intercept the march on Rome of the legionaries fired on them and wounded Garibaldi himself.

After Aspromonte many former Garibaldi legionaries who were serving in the regular Italian army resigned their commissions. This was due partly to the suspicious attitude of the government, understandably uneasy about officers who might—and did— desert at any time to heed the call of Garibaldi to some new expedition. It was due partly also to the legionaries themselves who after years spent in the excitement of conspiracies and revolts had developed into a cross between the knight errant and the adventurer and had found the life of routine and discipline of a regular army unbearably dull. Some of them went to London to seek passage to America in order to enlist in the Federal Army during the Civil War or in the army of the Mexican republicans after peace was restored in the United States. Mazzini, to whom they usually appealed for help, was exasperated by that exodus, feeling that their duty was to remain in Italy, ready to take the field against Austria at the first opportunity—with the king, without the king, and even against the king.

It is obvious that Mazzini's interest in the Civil War first, and in the Mexican revolution later, though real, was subordinated to the overpowering idea of complete Italian unification. The Italians, he felt, by fighting their battle on their home ground would fight the same Hydra of slavery and tyranny which was rearing its many heads in various parts of the world; hence a victory for freedom in Italy would be a victory for the abolitionists in America and the republicans in Mexico as well. It is not surprising, therefore, to find that there are few references in Mazzini's writings to the Civil War and its leaders. Lincoln is mentioned only a few times, mostly in connection with his assassination; no comment is found on any of Lincoln's speeches or state papers, and there is no indication that Mazzini even read any of them.

A point of contact between Mazzini and Lincoln not appearing in the collected writings is the Italian translation attributed to Mazzini of a letter attributed to Lincoln. It has been claimed that in 1853 Lincoln wrote to the physicist Macedonio Melloni, Director of the Vesuvian Observatory, in answer to a request for an expression of opinion on the political reorganization of Europe which the Italian scientist had sent him through Faraday and Humboldt. The letter expresses complete sympathy with the ideals of European liberals and the national aspirations of Italians, Germans, and Irish for unity and independence of their respective countries. It also contains a forecast of the eventual disappearance of the two empires—the Austrian and the English—that hindered the realization of those aspirations. It sees the eventual liberation of the Irish from England, the unification of Germany, including Alsace, and the unification of Italy, including the three major islands, Malta, and the Dalmatian coast, and a future federation of Europe reorganized on the basis of nationality. To the letter is attached a note in which Mazzini states that it was a "literal translation of the message sent by Abraham Lincoln to Macedonio Melloni in 1853 from Springfield, Illinois, made from the original autograph . . . with eyes wet with tears and a full heart, at the request of Countess Fulvia Salazar di Promanengo."[13] Serious objections have been made against the authenticity of both the letter and the translation, and they have not been satisfactorily answered.

Another point of contact between Mazzini and Lincoln is the striking correspondence between a famous phrase in the most famous of Lincoln's speeches, the Gettysburgh Address, and a phrase in one of Mazzini's manifestoes published twelve years earlier. The phrase "government of the people, by the people, for the people," corresponds almost word for word with Mazzini's "Republique du Peuple, par le Peuple et pour le Peuple," which occurs at the close of the "Manifesto of the European Democratic Committee to the Italians" in which Mazzini, explaining the meaning and implications of the motto *God and the People*, asks the question: "What does it mean if not a living equality, in other words, republic of the people, by the people, and for the people?" (*46* : 104).

Scholars have found a large number of analogues of this famous phrase in English and American literature and oratory. Similar expressions were used by Patrick Henry, Thomas Cooper, and John Adams in the eighteenth century, and in the nineteenth century by the British James Douglas, Lord John Russell, George Thompson, and by the Americans Chief Justice Marshall, President Monroe, Daniel Webster, Lieutenant M. F. Maury, Senator Henry Wilson, and Dr. Theodore Parker. To Parker seems to belong the honor of having suggested the expression to Lincoln, since the analogues found in Parker's sermons and pamphlets were read and underlined with pencil by Lincoln. A few analogues have also been found in continental European literature: in a speech by Schinz, a Swiss orator, in Friedrich Karl von Savigny's *System of Contemporary Roman Law*, and in Lamartine's *History of the Girondists*.[14]

Besides these well-known analogues, some not so well known can be found in other continental writers. The French statesman and historian L. A. Thiers in 1830 wrote in the prospectus of the newspaper *National*: "If we do not succeed in disciplining a hereditary power to the laws of the government of the country by the country, we shall seek beyond the Atlantic the model of a responsible elective power, completely submitted and enchained to the national will."[15]

The phrase "government of the country by the country" must have struck Mazzini, because he employed it two years later to define his idea of popular sovereignty in a letter to the Swiss historian Sismondi outlining the program of the newly founded Young Italy. "Here is the germ of all we shall attempt to develop later on: republican system, unitarian in so far as compatible with the greatest possible extent given to communal and municipal liberties; popular government, or, if you prefer, government of the country by the country." (*3* : 18).

Similar expressions kept on recurring through the years in Mazzini's writings. This is not surprising if we recall that to Mazzini *vox populi, vox Dei* was not a rhetorical expression but a literal truth. The myth "people" occupied in his political system the same cardinal place that "humanity" held in his religion, namely, that of revealer of divine truth to the individual man. Here are a few of the quotations that can be gleaned from his writings:

1831   ... may they be cursed for the peoples and by the peoples! (*2* : 13)
            Revolutions are made for the people and by the people. (*2* : 68)
1832   Revolutions must be made *for the people and by the people*. (*2* : 166, 189)
1833   Young Italy ... conceives as revolutions only those that are made in the name of the people, for the people, and by the people. Those alone are great, just, and lasting. (*3* : 341)
1834   The liberty of all must be conquered by all. (*4* : 177)
1838   Those who maintain ... *All through the People and all for the People*—maintain it precisely because they believe the People alone can accomplish all for the people. (*17* : 258)
            The people are seldom ungrateful or suspicious of virtuous intelligence. ... We ask no other proof, in modern times, than the consecutive ability that has been called to the Presidency of

the United States. Intelligence will govern through the people
and for the people. (*17* : 259)

1846 We have torn the great and beautiful ensign of democracy: *the
progress of all, through all, under the leadership of the best and wisest.*
(*34* : 100)

1849 Independence, that is the destruction of the internal and external
obstacles which hinder national life, must be achieved . . . not
only for the people but by the people. Battle of all, victory of
all. (*39* : 342)

1851 What does it mean if not a living Equality, in other words,
Republic of the People, by the People, and for the People?
(46 : 104)

1858 The rising of Italy must be the work of all and progress of all.
(*62* : 28)

1870 The Republic—government of all, by means of all, and for the
benefit of all. (*88* : 309)

We may add to the above quotations from Mazzini one from Kossuth's speech delivered before the Ohio Legislature at Columbus
on February 6, 1852, in which he stated: "The spirit of our age is
Democracy. All for the people and all by the people. Nothing
about the people without the people."[16] Mazzini reported also the
publication of a manifesto by a German liberal group bearing on
its masthead the motto, "All for the people, all by means of the
people" (*62* : 375).

Without attempting the hopeless and useless task of tracing
derivations and influences, it is safe to conclude that when Lincoln
gave utterance and prominence to the expression "government
of the people, by the people, for the people" the slogan was a
familiar one among liberal thinkers on both sides of the Atlantic.
Indeed, the reason the popularity of the slogan endured was exactly that it was not a formula conceived by a solitary thinker but
rather a pithy expression defining the ideal of popular sovereignty
and popular government that all the people of the Western world
were striving to realize.

CHAPTER X

THE UNIVERSAL REPUBLICAN ALLIANCE

THE PLAN of an alliance between the United States and the European republicans first proposed to Lincoln during the Civil War was again revived by Mazzini as soon as peace was restored in America. This time, however, instead of approaching men in official position he decided to appeal to leading individuals in their private capacity. The first to whom he broached the subject, and the first whose aid he sought, was Moncure Daniel Conway, the Unitarian minister previously mentioned. Conway had gone to London in 1862 on a propaganda tour for the Union financed by the Boston review *Commonwealth*, of which he was the editor, and by a group of friends—Emerson among them. In 1863, at the completion of his tour Conway decided to accept a call from the Unitarian South Place Chapel, Finsbury, London, and filled that pulpit until 1884. He remained in close contact with America and was, for a time at least, the London correspondent of the *New York Tribune* and a contributor to the *Commonwealth* and other American periodicals.

Thinking that as the correspondent of an important liberal daily Conway could help him by writing of his plan to his friends in America, Mazzini addressed a letter to him on May 25, 1865, in which he gave the broad outline of the plan. The ideas expressed follow the familiar Mazzini pattern: every nation has a mission, a special function, a peculiar role to play in the family of nations, without which it has no right to exist as such. The American mission was to uphold the republican principle not only within its own boundaries but everywhere in the world. This duty also coincided with enlightened self-interest, because the supporters of the antithetical principle, the monarchical, were already leagued together against the republicans, and had already set up an out-post in Mexico right at the back door of the United States. For her own sake as well as for the sake of the principle she repre-sented America had to take action; she had to intervene in Mexico immediately and, at the same time, enable the European republic-ans to attack simultaneously Austria and France. For their action the republicans needed some assistance—a modest sum, thirty to fifty thousand dollars, and a steam frigate.

Conway refused to give any coöperation. "With my abhorrence of war," he related in his *Autobiography*, "I could not expouse his [Mazzini's] scheme for European conflagration with the United States for participant, and his letter of May 25, 1865, was not communicated to any one."[1] But a few months later he requested of Mazzini an expression of opinion on the question of suffrage for the emancipated Negroes, a question which was being debated in America, and Mazzini took that occasion to repeat once again his arguments in favor of the alliance between republicans in America and in Europe. The controversial question of Negro suffrage had to be settled, he felt, so that America could stand united for the fulfillment of her mission—the leadership of the republicans of the world. She had to take her post "in the great battle being fought the world over between good and evil, justice and injustice, equality and privilege, duty and egoism, republic and monarchy, truth and falsehood, God and the idols." Her first task was to destroy that "outpost of Caesarism"—the Mex-ican Empire—established along her own frontiers (*83* : 163–67).

When the less than lukewarm attitude of Conway convinced him that no contact with liberal Americans could be made through him, Mazzini decided to send a representative to America to present his plan directly. He consulted a number of French and Polish refugees. Ledru-Rollin and a few others were sceptical about its success, but he insisted, and a Polish refugee, Louis Bulewski, was chosen to carry the message to America.

Supplied with numerous letters of introduction to "good liber-al advanced men" from Peter and Clementia Taylor, Conway, and others whom Clementia was able to enlist, Bulewski sailed for New York at the end of 1865 and set to work to line up support for Mazzini's scheme. He visited Washington and received some encouragement from several members of Congress.[2] When sufficient support was assured, a public meeting was held in New

York (April 19, 1866) at the Loyal Publication Rooms, 813 Broadway, "for the purpose of listening to an address to the friends of the republican principles in America, from the Republicans in Europe." There Bulewski read the following address by Mazzini.

If it is true that duties are proportionate to power, new duties rise today for the United States. The power of the United States, not only in the great American continent but also in Europe—after the war and the abolition of slavery—is immense. You have the power, hence you have the duty to be a leading and initiating country. And in order to perform such a duty you only need to represent the principle of your national life within and without your geographical boundaries.

The principle of your life is the republican principle, the principle toward which tends progressive Europe, and which either openly or latently, determines all European struggles.

Throughout Europe, and beyond Europe, a great struggle is taking place between the States constituted by Kings in the most arbitrary manner, and Nationalities defined by the needs and aspirations of the people; between republican faith and monarchical interests. You must come forward and take your place in the battle. It is God's battle.

A nation lives a twofold life—internal and external—manifestations of the same principle in two different spheres. There is a period—historically the first in the life of a people—during which a Nation must necessarily be concerned exclusively in constituting itself. For you this period is complete today. The vitality and the strength of your country were lately proven beyond any doubt. A new period begins for you. You are called by the admiration, by the sympathies, by the expectation of all progressive Europe, to affirm your essence before kings and peoples, to assume an office for the general progress of Humanity. The monarchical powers are federated to promote their interests. It is time now that, abandoning a system of isolation which involves an unworthy sentiment of inferiority, the republicans everywhere bind themselves into an alliance. It is ours not a faith? and is not every faith essentially propaganda? Moreover, the alliance of which we speak is not only a duty and a glorious office for the United States, but a necessity, a defensive measure.

Enough to consider Mexico. The bold step taken by Louis Napoleon there, is only the beginning of an aggressive policy that will not be abandoned by dynastic Europe. This policy has already attracted Spain; it is striving, though in vain, to attract England. You are too powerful, hence are feared as a danger; therefore you may rest assured that European despotism will not fail to attempt to weaken, harm, dismember you, if possible. Will you allow despotism to choose the time and place of the attack? Even in such a case, and alone, without a doubt you would win, but with serious sacrifice of American blood, which should be spared, and American gold, which should be put to better use. By means of a timely fraternal alliance with the European republican party you could avoid the danger, strike the evil at its root, and fulfill your sacred mission toward Europe, by promoting the triumph of Right, Truth, Justice, and laying the foundation of a new moral, political, and commercial era for your country. Old States will disappear and new Nations will rise to life; and these new nations will recognize with special bonds of gratitude, the aid they received from you in their days of trial. Should these views meet with your approval, our envoy will explain to you our aspirations, hopes, and desires (*83* : 187–89).

After the reading of the address, on a motion by Mr. E. A. Stansbury a special committee of five was appointed by the president, Col. F. A. Conklin, to draft a reply. The committee was further directed to circularize the reply for signatures, to give it publicity in the press, and to take all other steps deemed necessary to establish a more permanent organization of the association. The *New York Tribune* commented favorably on the appeal in an editorial which concluded that the "proposition of the London Committee is one of great importance, and only needs to be fully understood to meet everywhere with cordial approbation and moral support."[3] Two months later a similar meeting was held in Boston for the same purpose.[4] At about the same time the response of the New York committee was published with an impressive array of signatures. The signatures included the names of six U.S. Senators: Wilson of Massachusetts, Howard of Michigan, Wade of Ohio, Doolittle of Wisconsin, Ramsey of Minnesota, and Nye of Nevada, thirty-four members of the House of Representatives, mostly from the middlewest, and a number of prominent liberals such as William C. Bryant, Horace Greely, Henry J. Raymond, Gerrit Smith, and Thurlow Weed.

But if the number and the eminence of the signers was encouraging, the tenor of the response was too cautious and diplomatic to justify any excess of enthusiasm on the part of Mazzini and his friends. It began by reassuring the European brethren that the Americans had not weakened their national devotion to human rights. They were fully conscious of the increased responsibility that went with their increased power. They looked with more interest than ever on the efforts of Europeans to improve their political conditions. They were aware of the violation of the principle of nonintervention committed in the American continent by the very powers who enunciated and defined that doctrine. The response added that America would never tolerate the imposition of a dynastic rule on a territory conterminous with its own and assured the European brethren that "in this impregnable fortress of freedom raised by the millions, and consecrated by their suffering and blood" the Americans "will cherish sympathy and collect support" for nations oppressed by arbitrary rules. It pointedly stated, however, that Americans were mindful of the duty of all countries to keep "the sacred obligations of National neutrality," and that such a duty was enjoined upon them by the even "higher sanction" of the farewell words of Washington advising them to have as little political connection as possible with foreign countries and by Jefferson's dictum on "entangling alliances." "These words indicate an inviolable rule of personal obligation to refrain from every act liable to charge our government with an infraction of neutrality." As private individuals only, "heeding well the dignity, and careful of the honor of their government," they responded to the appeal, promised to extend the association over the whole country, and expressed the hope "that ere long the American voice will reach you in the assuring tones of American liberty."[5]

Though the response was not as enthusiastic as he had hoped, Mazzini felt that he had succeeded "to a certain extent," and he was glad that the attempt was made "against the discouraging vote of Ledru-Rollin and others," because it was a "germ of good for the future" (*82* : 110, 200). And he set about immediately to draft a detailed plan for the organization of the alliance in America and for its relations with the European counterpart.

The plan suggested by Mazzini followed the usual pattern of all Mazzini's associations: organization from above, arrangements for a journal, and sale of "bonds" to collect contributions. For the recruiting of members he counseled the organizers "to centralize in a chosen point, under a chosen and inspiring body, the whole of the organization" and "to establish . . . a Central Committee in every State, sub-committees in every town of some importance." For the press he advised that the publication of a republican paper in monarchical Europe would encounter so many insurmountable difficulties that it would be preferable to publish instead a series of pamphlets numbered consecutively, bearing the heading "Universal Republican Alliance." These pamphlets published in French at irregular times and different places would be immediately translated for the different national sections of the alliance into their respective languages. The American committee could contribute either manuscript essays or printed material they wished to have circulated in Europe. Finally, for the finances he suggested the issuance of subscription notes of one, five, ten, and twenty dollars to be bought by the members upon joining according to their means and liberality. A certain percentage of the proceeds would be remitted to the European committee. A specimen of these notes was sent to the American committee in New York. It showed two ladies in Frigian cap (Europe and America) standing on opposite shores of the ocean, one of them holding the staff and the other the free end of a flag bearing the legend "Universal Republican Alliance" (*86* : 69–77).[6]

At the same time, upon the suggestion of Bulewski, Mazzini wrote to Gerrit Smith explaining the financial arrangements submitted to the American committees and requesting his support for this tie between Europe and America, or, as he called it, "the laying of the moral Atlantic Cable" (*82* : 288–92).

Gerrit Smith, a wealthy landowner and philanthropist with radical views in both politics and religion, had been identified for over thirty years with numerous reform movements—abolition of slavery, equal rights for women, temperance movement, free soil movement, and so on. He had long been an admirer of Mazzini, and fifteen years earlier, on November 14, 1851, after reading one of his articles in a British paper, had addressed a letter to him replete with expressions of admiration and love.[7] The following year at the time of Kossuth's tour, in a letter to Frederick Douglass he called Mazzini "a wise and profound philosopher," and expressed the hope that he too would visit America, feeling sure that "he would . . . make broader and more effective appeals to our human nature than Kossuth has done."[8]

He was exceedingly pleased when Bulewski called on him to deliver Mazzini's letter. "I have long honored and loved you," he replied, "regarding you as one of the truest and sublimest interpreters of the Divine Will, and one of the bravest and wisests leaders of our poor humanity in its upward struggle from the abyss of ignorance and superstition, and in its repeated endeavors now here, now there, to escape the crushing folds of despotism." He agreed heartily with Mazzini's plan of alliance between republicans of the Old and the New World, and declared that Americans ought to give their European brethren an aid of at least fifty to one hundred thousand dollars a year.[9]

Mazzini may have felt encouraged by this letter, especially if Bulewski informed him of the generosity with which Smith was accustomed to aid the causes he believed in. But his hopes were soon dimmed by the fact that he did not hear further from Smith and by the silence with which the New York and Boston committees greeted his suggested plan of organization.

Mazzini found this silence and evident inactivity particularly disconcerting because just about that time he had decided to resume openly his republican propaganda in Italy. After the campaigns of 1859 and 1860 and the resulting proclamation of the Kingdom of Italy, Mazzini had tacitly accepted the will of the people, and had refrained from any direct propaganda and conspiratorial activity against the new regime. He had confined himself to theoretical propaganda in favor of republican institutions conducted subtly, by "teaching republicanism by contrast," as he termed it, "mainly by showing in articles on America, Switzerland, etc., the superiority of the system" (67 : 224–25) or by "praising America compared to despotism and bastard constitutionalism" (67 : 250). He followed this line of conduct until the Summer of 1866. The outcome of the war between Italy and Prussia on one side, and Austria on the other side, filled him with disgust. He had put his light of republicanism under a bushel for the sake of Italy's unity. To achieve that unity, albeit a monarchical unity, he had postponed indefinitely his dream of a republic, and now he saw that the fruit of the sacrifice of the republicans was the shame of Custozza and Lissa and the humiliation of receiving Venice from the hands of Napoleon. The monarchists had persisted in the policy of distrust of the people. They had revealed during the war their unwillingness to arm the volunteers and to encourage a Venetian revolt against Austria. It was a policy that had resulted in the defeat and dishonor of the country. He appealed to Garibaldi to lead a protest against the humiliating peace, and when Garibaldi declined, he appealed to the people with the "Manifesto of the Republican Alliance" in which he reviewed all past and present grievances against the Savoy monarchy and stated the reasons why the republicans had to break the truce and take up again their work of agitation.[10]

It was therefore important to Mazzini to have the American organization in working order, both for the financial help he hoped to obtain and for the propaganda value its existence would have for the work in Italy. He decided to stimulate the American committees into activity with another emissary, this time William J. Linton, the English journalist, artist, reformer, who was already well known in American liberal circles. He had been closely associated with American liberals for over twenty years. Since Linton was going to the United States at the end of 1866, Mazzini entrusted him with the task of reorganizing the alliance. He gave him letters of introduction to the presidents of the New York and Boston committees and to Gerrit Smith and a set of directives which summarized what had been accomplished and outlined the work still to be done. The directives included the following:

At the beginning of the year, I proposed an organized Alliance between European and American Republicans. My address was answered, rather cautiously by the New York Committee, very warmly by the Boston one. The bearer of my proposal was Bulewski. He came back with plenty of encouragement and written promises.

I was asked to propose the first steps. I did so. I proposed that Committees and sub-committees of the Alliance should be organized everywhere through the States;—that tickets of admission, subscription notes, should be published worth one, five, ten, twenty dollars, and that each member should choose one as document of his belonging to the Alliance—that a certain part of the result should come to us for the purpose of promoting morally and materially our republican aim, and a certain part remain in the United States for the purpose of spreading the principles of the Republican Alliance—that the notes of which I sent a sample should have at the top "Universal Republican Alliance," symbols representing America and Europe, and three signatures for the Alliance: Ledru-Rollin's, my own, and an American—that from the United States there should come to us pamphlets, articles, tracts putting the American questions in the proper light, to be published or re-published by us; and that we should send pamphlets, articles, documents on our own questions, to be translated and published in America—and so on.

To these proposals I have never had any answer. They promised again, explained the delay as coming from the absorbing internal question, etc., but the delay has been prolonging itself to the actual day.

Your object must therefore be to urge them to realize the scheme practically or to ascertain that nothing can be done. You will urge them, describing the actual moment as the one to be chosen—the moral fall of Louis Napoleon in France, the prestige gone, the failures in Mexico, in Prussia, in England about the Congress, in Italy and everywhere, having acted on the French mind—the illness, the possible sudden death, and the intention of the republicans—the Eastern question afloat—the increase, especially since the late war, of the Republican Party in Italy, the possibility of a rising, the Roman question opening in December next, the only objection in Italy to a change being the fear of a monarchical Europe being against, the importance therefore of a material help and of any moral sympathy manifested from the United States to us—the possibility of yielding to the United States some naval station if wanted on the Dalmatian shore on the Adriatic, or of commercial compacts.

The language of the Press exhorting us to a Republic—a certain number of revolving rifles—a contact between me and the diplomatic agents of the United States in Italy—means of corresponding safely through them in Rome—money for both Italy and the French workingmen-associations—these and other things would be of importance to us.

You must advert to the position of Spain where the regime is now such as to make a revolution not only possible but probable. And advert to the importance of the religious question in Rome.

Stansbury and Claffin are the Presidents of the New York and Boston Committees. Should you, by chance, not find them, Col. Rush C. Hawkins, Bible House, New York, and Judge Thomas Russell, 35 Court Street, Boston, are the Secretaries. The letters may be delivered to them (*84* : 75–80).

On his arrival in New York, Linton realized that his task was not merely to awaken the committees, which in reality no longer existed, but to do the work all over again. He wrote to Mazzini (December 6, 1866) explaining the situation. He outlined a new plan of organization and requested him to send a delegation of power to act in the name of the alliance. Mazzini did so, cautioning his friend to avoid giving offense to the members of the defunct committees and advising him to see personally at least two of them, Gerrit Smith and G. L. Stearns (*84* : 181–85).

In January, Linton had two documents printed in New York under the name of "The Universal Republic." One was a scheme of organization which stated that the object of the association was "to maintain the right of every Country to a Republican Government, and the consequent duty of all Republicans to unite for a solidarity of Republics." All liberal and freethinking men were to unite in national associations, each of which would constitute a "republic . . . of the present or of the future." Each of these "republics" was to elect a secretary to represent them in a central council, consisting, in addition to the delegates of the several associations, of a president, a financial secretary, and a recording secretary. "These branches, being kept distinct, will stand as representative republics, while their delegates, forming a Central Council, will represent the Solidarity of Republics, for the realization of which, in actual government, the association is pledged to labor." The publications sponsored by the association were to be under the authority of a special committee appointed by the central council. The funds to be devoted to the European work were to be placed at the disposal of Mazzini.

The other document was a pledge to be signed by the applicant, a sort of creed of the association, which read:

I believe in the REPUBLIC—the organization of a free people on the ground of equal political and social rights—as the only means through which a nation may be enabled to will and act, as one man, for the fulfillment of its own destiny and the accomplishment of its duty to Humanity.

And as I believe in the necessity of republican organization for a single nation in order that it may obtain its full growth and completeness, I am compelled to believe in the necessity of republican organization for all the nations of the world; so I believe in the solidarity of Humanity, the duty of nation toward nation, and the duty of every individual in every nation not only to his nation but to the world;

I believe, therefore, that it is the right and bounded duty of every nation and of every man to aid to the utmost the striving of other nations or of other men toward the establishment of the Universal Republic;

And I pledge myself as a member of this Association to the best of my ability and means to aid in the propagation and practical realization of this my belief.[11]

Following Mazzini's suggestion, Linton wrote to Gerrit Smith to inform him that nothing had been done since the departure of Bulewski and that he was endeavoring to "quietly enroll names, and as soon as we number enough to assure a good public meeting, then to organize publicly the association."[12] But although Linton on that occasion remained in America for six months, he must never have obtained enough pledges, because no public meeting was held.

The return of Linton to England in June, 1867, marked the end of the attempt to organize the Universal Republican Alliance in America. Even Gerrit Smith—who was enthusiastic about the undertaking and who, on reading the manifesto of the alliance in the *Atlantic Monthly* had written to Mazzini saluting him as "Dear friend of God and Man" and mailed a contribution of five hundred dollars—signed the pledge but never mailed it because there was no organization to receive it.

In spite of this failure the organization of the alliance in America was often mentioned by Mazzini in his propaganda in Europe, especially in Italy. He had the documents printed by Linton in America published in friendly newspapers in Italy (*84* : 223, 224, 251, 256). He pointed to the progress of the alliance in North America to urge Cuneo to organize a branch in South America (*84* : 219, 220, 249–50). He assured Giuseppe Nathan and Gennaro Bovio in Italy that the association was "widespread in the United States," "that it has deep roots in the United States of America, and will have powerful public development as soon as the conflict between the President and the Congress will cease absorbing the activity of American republicans" (*85* : 227–28, 306).

But Mazzini's efforts were no more successful in Europe than they had been in America. There was a Polish center of the alliance in Lousanne and an Italian chapter at Lugano which may have never progressed beyond the appointment of committees. The only locality where the alliance achieved a widespread organization was Sicily, where it was closely watched by the Italian government. On a visit that Mazzini attempted there to contact the leaders personally, he was promptly arrested and whisked away to the fortress of Gaeta and detained for several weeks.

It is curious to note that the "Fundamental Statute of the Universal Republican Alliance" was published in Italy only in October, 1868, almost three years after the first attempt to organize the association in America. The statement of principle in the preamble goes far in explaining why the movement failed to achieve any degree of success.

The Universal Republican Alliance is composed of all those citizens who, recognizing that the Monarchy is the sole and real cause of the misfortunes of the people, profess firm and sincere faith in the republican principle. Therefore those who believe impossible the realization of the republican government in Italy, and the formation of the United States of Europe as a foundation to the universal brotherhood of all people, cannot be members of this Association. The Universal Republican Alliance is unitarian for Italy; it wants to become an armed corps, and is connected and bound with a brotherly pact with all the free peoples of the earth.

The Republican Alliance therefore has for its aim in the political field, the hastening of the triumph of the Republican Unity of Italy, the winning of her natural boundaries, of all its provinces subject to foreign domination, and the proclamation at the earliest moment of the Republic—as a signal of universal brotherhood.

In the social order it asserts the equality of all citizens; it opposes therefore all privileges of cast, it does not recognize any inequality of rights and duties before the law, which must be the expression of the majority, with its basis in morality and justice. Consequently it advocates universal suffrage, free from all limitations.

In the economic field it fights for the complete emancipation of the proletariat from the tyranny of capital, advocating cooperation instead of present day wages, so that capital may become an associate of labor (*86* : 169–70).

It was a program not substantially different from that offered by Young Italy thirty-six years before, and it failed to have a wide appeal at that late date because the issues it raised were either dead or were no longer the exclusive property of the republicans. Italy was united and independent; the achievement of "natural" boundaries was advocated with equal fervor by all political parties; the institutional question of republic versus monarchy had lost relevance for the Italians because most of them felt there was no political, social, or economic reform they could not carry out under a constitutional monarchy equally as well as under a republic; and, finally, on the more vital economic issue, Mazzini's vague opposition to the "tyranny of capital" was no longer strong enough to make Italians deaf to the siren song of the new reformers, Bakunin and Marx, who promised a more facile and prompt realization of the aspirations of the proletariat. Mazzini had accomplished his own peculiar task, his "mission," so well that he was no longer needed, and he was, in his last years, admired and revered by all but heeded by none.

CHAPTER XI

CONCLUSION

~~~~~~

FROM A PRACTICAL standpoint Mazzini's connections with America resolved themselves into a succession of failures. His relations with the Christian Alliance in the forties, Young America in the fifties, the Universal Republican Alliance in the sixties, did not achieve anything concrete. The organizations he set up or inspired in America—Young Italy, the Committee for European Democracy, the Action Party, the Republican Alliance—all had an ephemeral existence. His drive for funds in the United States, like those of the German Kinkel and the Hungarian Kossuth, never netted more than trifling amounts.

But before dismissing Mazzini as a failure for not achieving what he set out to do, one should examine the question whether his influence did not transcend his insuccess. Mazzini failed in Italy. Unification there was achieved in a manner and by means different from, and even in contrast with, what he proposed. Still, Italian unification, however achieved, would have been inconceivable without his tireless propaganda and conspiratorial activity that knew no discouragement, that acknowledged no defeat, that ceaselessly haunted tyrants and weaklings, and that precluded any other solution for the Italian problem but that of national unity. It is true that it took the genius of Cavour to steer a course clear of the reefs of domestic contrasts and the shoals of international intrigues. But this Cavour could do only after Mazzini had created at home the passionate longing for unity and abroad the fear that unless Italy were united by a monarch it would be united by the "red republicans." Cavour could gather the scattered limbs of Italy only after Mazzini had made it one in spirit.

So it was with his influence abroad. In England he was never the object of popular acclaim like Kossuth in 1851 and Garibaldi in 1864. His influence was always limited to small groups in which women were usually so prominent that someone could scornfully refer to his English following as "a half a dozen skirts." Still, his influence on English thought, it is generally conceded, was greater than that of any other foreigner, no matter how popular temporarily. This writer is not prepared to state that the same is true for America. But he cannot help wondering how deep his influence must have reached into the American soil when he reads of Jane Addams' father grief stricken in his Illinois farmhouse at the news of Mazzini's death or of Dr. Herron's childhood in a Quaker community in Indiana which had a sort of religious devotion for the Italian leader.[1]

Before the Civil War, Mazzini looked with interest and sympathy upon the American republic, though at first his admiration was somewhat dampened by the existence of slavery and by the emphasis on individual rights at the expense of the welfare of the group. The republics of the future, he thought, would be more authoritarian and religious than the United States (*32* : 221). But in spite of this reservation, he assigned to the United States, together with Switzerland, the task of teaching the world "the practical application of the republican form of government" (*46* : 220–21); and to the United States, alone among non-European countries, he assigned a civilizing role outside its boundaries, especially in Mexico and South America, where, "the American Anglo-Saxons will give humanity better contributions than those given by the Ibero-Latin race, or the copper colored tribes" (*62* : 311–12).

After the Civil War he saw America in a still more exalted role. America, cleansed of the pollution of slavery, strong with the power revealed in the long and bloody struggle between the states, had no longer the somewhat passive role of teacher of republicanism but that of leader of the liberal forces of the world. In other words, the role that America eventually had to accept almost a century later was envisioned by Mazzini in a letter to Conway dated October 30, 1865.

With a sum of force almost fabulous in energy unknown to our monarchies; through the constant devotion of your men and women, and the indomitable courage of your improvised soldiers; and above all thanks to the obliteration of slavery—the only blot that sullied your glorious republican standard—you have impressed in the heart of Europe the conviction that in you abides a force, a power almost incal-

culable, at the service of human progress. The numerous and ever
growing republican elements in Europe have discovered in you their
representative. You have become a Nation-Guide, and you must act as
such. In the great battle being fought the world over between good and
evil, justice and injustice, equality and privilege, duty and egoism,
republic and monarchy, truth and falsehood, God and the idols, your
place is marked and you must take it.

As workers for Humanity you must feel that standing aloof is a crime;
that indifference, when the cry of a human creature calls you, is atheism....
You must manfully aid morally and, if necessary, materially your republican brethren everywhere the sacred battle is fought. You can
encourage and strengthen those who suffer and bleed for truth and
justice. This is your mission; this is your glory and safety; this is your
future! (*83* : 166–67).

APPENDICES · NOTES · INDEX

UNPUBLISHED LETTER OF GERRIT SMITH TO MAZZINI

~~~~~~

Transcript courteously supplied by Mr. Lester G. Wells, Curator of the Gerrit Smith Miller Collection at the Syracuse University Library.

<div align="right">

Peterboro, State of New York
Nov. 14, 1851

</div>

JOSEPH MAZZINI,

It is a plain and private individual who presumes to address you. That I am not an impostor, you might know, if it were necessary for you to know so unimportant a thing, by inquiring of Joseph Sturge of Birmingham, or John Scoble of London, who is Secretary of the British and Foreign Anti Slavery Society, or George Thompson, member of the British Parliament.

The occasion of my writing you this letter is my joy in reading in a late British Newspaper an Essay from your pen in which you speak of "the fatal separation between religious and political belief;" and of its being "necessary to reunite earth to Heaven,—politics to the eternal principles, which should direct them."

Such sentiments, as these, have warmed my heart for many years. In my feeble way I have sought to inculcate them. I am a member of a small political party (Liberty Party) which cherishes and acts upon them.

You will learn something of the character of this Party by the speech which I herewith send you.

I love and honor you. I pray for God's blessing upon you. It would rejoice me to receive a few lines from your hand. Your bare autograph I should regard as a treasure. How much more were it accompanied by some of your noble sentiments!

<div align="right">

Your friend,
GERRIT SMITH

</div>

APPENDIX B

UNCOLLECTED LETTERS
OF MAZZINI

The following are letters which escaped the attention of the editors of Mazzini's *Scritti editi ed inediti*.

1. TO GEORGE N. SANDERS

In 1914, the papers of G. N. Sanders were sold at public auction by the American Art Association of New York. The catalogue of the sale listed eight letters from Mazzini, only one of which, No. 148, was later published in *Scritti* (*Appendix 5*: 219–20). The descriptions of the letters are reproduced below as they appear in the *Illustrated Catalogue of the political Correspondence of the late Hon. George N. Sanders, Confederate Commissioner to Europe during the Civil War* (New York, 1914).

144   Mazzini (Giuseppe)—Italian patriot, devoted himself to the liberation of Italy. A. L. S. (in English), 2 pp. 12mo. London, no date, but Feb., 1854 (to G. N. Sanders).
Interesting small letter, with mention of Kossuth, Felix Orsini, etc.

145   Mazzini (Giuseppe) A. L. S. (in English), 1 p. 12mo. Undated, but London, March 3, 1854 (To G. N. Sanders) with mention of Kossuth.

146   Mazzini (Giuseppe) A. L. S. (in English). 2 pp. 12mo. London April 14, 1854. (To G. N. Sanders). A letter of introduction saying the bearer is a friend and a patriot.

147   Mazzini (Giuseppe) 2 A. L. S. (one slightly imperfect), both in English, 1 and 2 pp. 12mo. London, July 20, 1854 (To G. N. Sanders). One contains mention of the Federal Council, etc.

148   Mazzini (Giuseppe) A. L. S. (in English), 2 pp. 12mo. No place, but London, April 18, 1857. (To G. N. Sanders). An interesting letter, with references to "the good cause for which I am fighting," etc.

149   Mazzini (Giuseppe). A. L. S. (in English) 6 pp. 12mo. No place, Jan. 15, 1858 (To G. N. Sanders).

156

Letter commences "My dear Friend," "Am I forgotten by you, I hope not ... I beg to recommend to you one of my friends, Captain Augustus Elia of Ancona ... one of our most devoted patriots ... [then follows account of a visit from Kossuth, etc.] ... I am in England now ... I do still believe that we ought to find your help from a few wealthy American sympathizers ... but I have no hopes ... still, I do firmly believe that America would be more benefited in her future mission ... than by any other thing you now attempt," etc.

150 Mazzini (Giuseppe). A. L. S. (in English), 2 pp. 12mo. No place, but London, April 18, 1858. (To Mrs. G. N. Sanders).
"... Italy ... from whence I come back ... more pledged than ever to our flag," etc.

151 Mazzini (Giuseppe). A. L. S. (in English), 3 pp. 12mo. (portion cut away from two pages). No place, but London, August 5, 1858. (To G. N. Sanders). Also an A. L. S. of Fed. Campanella, Mazzini's secretary, to G. N. Sanders. Together, 2 pieces.

2. To Theodore Dwight Weld

The following letter was published in the *Liberator* of April 22, 1859, as a "letter from Mazzini ... received a few days ago by the Principal of a private school in the vicinity of New York." It was reprinted in the *National Era*, VIII (May 12, 1859), 76, and, in part, in W. S. Garrison, *Joseph Mazzini, his Life, Writings, and Political Principles* (New York, 1872), Intro pp. xvi-xvii. In no case was the identity of the "Principal" disclosed. There is no doubt, however, that the recipient was Theodore D. Weld, as shown by the context of the letter and the following item in the *New York Tribune* (Jan. 19, 1859): "Madame Mario addressed the pupils of Theodore Weld 'Eagleswood School' day before yesterday, upon the question of Italian Freedom. At the close of her discourse a collection amounting to $112 was taken among the boys and the girls, to be remitted to London for the benefit of Mazzini's school."

London, March 21, 1859

Dear Sir:—I beg to apologize for being so late in acknowledging the receipt of $112.09, subscribed by you and others at the end of the lecture delivered at your institution by my friend, Mme Jessie M. White Mario, toward our Italian school, etc.

I am very much pleased at my honored friend's first success and response to her efforts in the United States, coming from Young America, to whom Young Italy looks for sympathy and support in her approaching struggle, and my thanks are the thanks of all the members, both teachers and pupils, of our Italian school.

We are fighting the same sacred battle for freedom and the emancipation of the oppressed,—you, Sir, against *negro*, we against *white* slavery. The cause is truly identical; for, depend upon it, the day in which we shall succeed in binding to one freely accepted pact twenty-six million of Italians, we shall give what we cannot now, an active support to the cause you pursue. We are both the servants of the God who says, "Before Me there is no Master, no Slave, no Man, no Woman, but only Human Nature, which must be everywhere responsible, therefore free."

May God bless your efforts and ours! May the day soon arrive in which the word BONDAGE will disappear from our living languages, and only point out a historical record! And, meanwhile, let the knowledge that we, all combatants under the same flag, do through time and space, commune in love and faith, strengthen one another against the unavoidable suffering which we must meet on the way. Believe me, my dear Sir,

Very gratefully yours,

Joseph Mazzini.

3. To Moncure Daniel Conway

This letter was published for the first time in M. D. Conway, *Autobiography* (Boston, 1904), II, 61–63. It is dated May 25, 1865.

Dear Mr. Conway,—The heroic struggle in your native land is at an end. Ought it not to be the beginning of a new era in American life?

The life of a great nation is twofold: inward and outward. A nation is a mission—a function in the development of mankind—or nothing. A nation has a task to fulfill in the world for the good of all, a principle it represents in a mighty struggle which constitutes history, a flag to hoist in the giant battle to which all local battles are episodes— going on in the earth between justice and injustice, liberty and tyranny, equality and arbitrary privilege, God and the devil. The non-interference doctrine is an atheistic one. To abstain is to deny the oneness of God and of mankind.

There is a time, a period, during which the implement must be fitted up, the *power* for action organized. The period requires *abstention*. You have gone through that period. It was right that the founders of the United States should say to them: "Abstain from all European concern." It would be mere selfism if they took that rule as a permanent one. You are now powerful with a *tested* power. You have asserted your *self*. You have, by the abolition of slavery, linked yourselves with the condition of Europe. The four years' list of noble deeds achieved by you all *must* be a christening to the great mission of which I speak. You have shown yourselves great: you have, therefore, great duties to perform.

You must represent the republican principle, which is your life, not only within your boundaries but everywhere, whenever it is possible to do so.

Europe—the republican Europe—expects you to do so. You *can* be a leading power amongst us; therefore you *ought* to be such a power.

All this is far higher than any consideration of safety. Still even *that* consideration is something. What you have done, and the applause of all struggling countries, have alarmed all the European monarchs. Depend upon it, they will not leave you at rest. The imperialist scheme, the Spanish scheme, the Austrian scheme, will go on. The Mexican affair is a programme.

You must interfere if you want to avoid being interfered with. You ought to grasp the opportunity. Your prestige is immense. You are in one of those decisive moments given by victory which was—on a smaller scale—before Garibaldi, after he had conquered Sicily and Naples. He might have achieved anything, had he not yielded to monarchies' bidding; you may *now* achieve anything.

League yourselves with our republican national parties. Let your representatives abroad be instructed to put themselves in contact with us and to give a word of encouragement to our efforts, a pledge of alliance with our future.

Go to Mexico: go quickly: insure a victory. Defeat the usurpers before they have reinforcements.

Let your proclamations say that you go, not for conquest's sake, but in the name of a principle, because you feel called to check the interfering progress of despotic monarchical schemes.

And help us to act *simultaneously* both in France and in Italy, against Austria and against the Empire, A sum of fifty, of thirty thousand dollars,—a steam-frigate sent—of course not officially—at our orders—will enable us to ensure triumph not only for ourselves, but for yourselves too.

Why am I saying this? Why do we not collect money in our own countries?

Of course we can. But it would take six months, one year. And everybody will know it. And every monarch will be on the alert. Now, if you go to Mexico, action on our side ought to be sudden and simultaneous.

I write these things to you, because you have friends in the United States to whom you may, perhaps, communicate these ideas, and who may find it advisable to embody them into facts. If so, the transaction ought to take place secretly and quickly.

Ever faithfully yours,

JOSEPH MAZZINI.

4. To WILLIAM LLOYD GARRISON

Published in W. L. Garrison, *Joseph Mazzini, his Life, Writings* (New York, 1872), Intro. p. xi.

My dear Friend,—We may never more see one another. Will you accept my photograph, and think of me sometimes? God bless you, and all those you love! Ever faithfully yours,

Jos. Mazzini

August 3, (1867), 18 Fulham Road, S. W.

APPENDIX C

INDEX OF AMERICANA IN MAZZINI'S WRITINGS

~~~~~~

This index lists references to America and Americans in Mazzini's *Scritti*. It includes also references found therein to Italians in America, but only for the duration of their American residence. An effort has been made to make this index as complete as possible. (All references are to the 100 volume *edizione nazionale*, *Scritti editi ed inediti* [Imola: Galeati, 1905–43]. Numerals in italics denote volumes; numerals in roman type, pages.)

ADAMS, Charles Francis: and Italian volunteers for Union Army, *73:* 347–48, 356

Agostini, L. E.: *Roma del Popolo* mailed to, *90:* 278

Albinola, Giovanni: member of New York chapter of Young Italy, *20:* 104; secretary of chapter, *20:* 262; *23:* 90; secretary of New York free school for poor Italians, *24:* 26; agent of Christian Alliance, *24:* 26

Alcott, Amos B. *23:* 220–21

America: no longer land of easy fortune, *15:* 431–32; as proof of triumph of republican principles, *20:* 50; as example of republicanism, *31:* 131; *67:* 224–25, 250; *86:* 205; *91:* 220; *92:* 104; as teacher of republicanism, *46:* 220–21; as world leader of republicanism, *83:* 165–67, 188–89; not sufficiently authoritarian and religious, *32:* 221; as example of tenacity, *93:* 184; high caliber of Presidents of, *17:* 259; civilizing mission of, *62:* 311–12; revolution unnecessary in, *66:* 266; militia in, *69:* 172; as example to Italy, *69:* 176, 345;

freedom of association in, *75:* 304; *93:* 217; *Appendix 4:* 235; popular initiative in, *83:* 349

—Aid from, *24:* 350; *25:* 283, 299– 300; *Appendix 2:* 286; certain, *50:* 28, 244; *60:* 378; *Appendix 3:* 62; hoped for, *24:* 10; *42:* 211; *44:* 235; *53:* 142; expected, *23:* 308; *47:* 145; *53:* 184; *56:* 41; necessary, *53:* 298; assured at start of revolution, *47:* 342–43; *Appendix 2:* 298; *Appendix 4:* 264; not received, *54:* 226–27, 329; stopped by Louis Napoleon's coup d'état, *47:* 317, 342–43; repaid with trade concessions, *58:* 34, and naval bases, *84:* 79. *See also* National Loan; War Chest

American Constitution: not suited to Italy, *26:* 87

American consul [unidentified]: in Marseilles, offers protection to Mazzini, *5:* 318, 363; at Malta, protests expulsion of Lemmi, *48:* 53; in London, gives Mazzini an American passport, *52:* 111; in London, to be given Mazzini's address, *72:* 283

161

American education: Mazzini requests information on, *71:* 244–45

American flag: flown at popular demonstration in Leghorn, *32:* 154–55

American Letters. See Mario, Jessie W.

American poetry: is "sickening," *60:* 182

American press: friendly to Mazzini's cause, *28:* 220–21

American Revolution: guerilla warfare in, *3:* 213; created American liberty, *8:* 351; similar to Milanese revolt, *36:* 248; as an example to Lombardy, *38:* 91, 216; as an example to Italy, *66:* 25, 264

American school [political], *6:* 348-49; *10:* 316, 326; *12:* 95; *19:* 425; *67:* 250; *77:* 48

Ancarani, R.: aids Alberto Mario in America, *61:* 299; supports Jessie W. Mario, *62:* 167–70; no longer in touch with Mazzini, *71:* 162; mentioned, *67:* 174

Angeloni, Luigi: advocates an Italian federation similar to the U.S.A., *14:* 251–52; *22:* 98

Apostolato: copies of, to America, *20:* 98, 262, 295; *23:* 333; *24:* 78, 106, 197, 382; *26:* 10–11; *28:* 220

Arese, Francesco: follows Louis Napoleon to America, *15:* 97

Argenti, Felice: deported to America, *11:* 124; holds funds of Italian war chest, *33:* 82; *35:* 43

Arms: for European revolution, *47:* 307; *51:* 251; possibility of buying, *52:* 174; deposits of, in the Mediterranean, *52:* 126–27, 318; *53:* 13; Kossuth urged to buy, *Appendix 4:* 163, 186–87, 210. See also Carbines

Atlantic Monthly: Mazzini sends article to, *85:* 12; is interested in an article in, *85:* 77; uncertain whether his article can be published by, *85:* 84; requested to write article on religious question in Italy for, *85:* 128

Attinelli, Giuseppe: teacher in the New York free school of Young Italy, *24:* 26

Avezzana, Giuseppe: member of Young Italy in New York, *20:* 104, 262; *33:* 53; letter to, *33:* 102–107; Mazzini re-established contact with,

42: 95; urged to organize Democrazia Europea in America, *44:* 64; member of Committee for National Italian Association, *44:* 77; requested to defend Mazzini, *44:* 167; aids Alberto Mario, *61:* 299; supports Jessie W. Mario, *62:* 167–170; protests against Piedmontese policy, *63:* 102; receives copy of Mazzini's *Parole, 65:* 374; *67:* 174; sends money draft, *67:* 213; separates from Mazzini, *71:* 162; aids New York free school of Young Italy, *77:* 272; recommended to Kossuth, *Appendix 4:* 162; receives copies of Mazzini's letter to Louis Napoleon, *Appendix 5:* 332; mentioned, *67:* 174; *68:* 106

BACHI, Pietro: founds Young Italy chapter in Boston, *20:* 104; opens free school for poor Italians, *23:* 73–74, 90; *77:* 272; Mazzini inquires about, *44:* 167; Alberto Mario must contact, *61:* 299

Bandiera Brothers: and American merchant marine, *26:* 177; medals in commemoration of, *27:* 42, 85; pamphlet on, *27:* 116, 134; *28:* 57

Bargnani, Alessandro: member of Young Italy in New York, *20:* 104, 262; agent of Christian Alliance in London, *28:* 129–30; brings letter for Confalonieri, *28:* 144; and Paris chapter of Young Italy, *28:* 176–77, 178–79, 182–83, 194, 203; is heard from, *28:* 248; Mazzini is in touch with, *40:* 289; goes to Liverpool, *Appendix 3:* 55. See also Christian Alliance

Bargnani, Gaetano: agent of Christian Alliance, *23:* 269–70; is to leave for Europe for Christian Alliance, *24:* 10. See also Christian Alliance

Barney, Hiram: and Jessie W. Mario, *61:* 66; *63:* 25, 29–30; Mazzini is disgusted with, *63:* 101

Bassini, Carlo: founds Young Italy chapter in Richmond, Va., *20:* 104; Mazzini inquires about, *44:* 167

Beecher, Henry Ward: member of committee sponsoring Jessie W. Mario in New York, *61:* 66

Beecher, Lyman: and Christian Alliance, *23:* 269

Bible societies: ineffective in Italy, *60:* 255–56. *See also* Christian Alliance

Biseo, Camillo: letters to, *67:* 173–74; *68:* 104–7; *71:* 162–64, 193–94; supports Jessie W. Mario, *62:* 167–70; *71:* 193; remittance from, *67:* 180, 233; Mazzini hears from, *67:* 265

Blind, Karl: requested to give Mazzini's address to American Consul, *72:* 283

Bonaccina, Giovan Maria: Mazzini inquires about, *44:* 167

Borsieri, Pietro: deported to America, *12:* 169

Boston, Mass.: Young Italy chapter founded in, *20:* 104; free school for poor Italians opened by Young Italy in, *23:* 73–74, 82, 90, 225; *24:* 88; *25:* 123, 160, 161; *77:* 272; Ferdinando Gori, Giovanni Galuzzi, Giuseppe Mussa expelled from Young Italy chapter in, *23:* 260, 268–69; Mazzini has no correspondents in, *68:* 107; Committee of Universal Republican Alliance in, *82:* 290; *84:* 181. *See also* Bachi, Pietro

Brown, John: as martyr to truth and justice, *76:* 34

Brown, Nicholas: Mazzini pleased with, *42:* 17; recommended to Mazzini's mother, *42:* 42, 48; urges Mazzini to refute slanders in American papers, *44:* 167; aids international correspondence of exiles, *50:* 204; asks Mazzini for report on execution of Ugo Bassi, *57:* 121

Brown, Mrs. Nicholas: introduced to F. Lamennais, *Appendix 4:* 82

Bruzzesi, G.: recommended to Siegel [Gen. Franz Sigel?], *72:* 351

Buchanan, James: withholds American passport of Italian exile, *54:* 209; and the Anglo-French navy in the Carribean, *62:* 362–63; not friendly to Mazzini, *Appendix 5:* 194–95

Bulewski, Louis: goes to London, *81:* 249; letters of introduction for, *81:* 261–62; not heard from, *81:* 295; as Mazzini's agent in America, *82:* 110; returns to London, *82:* 200; and Universal Republican Alliance,

84: 76; *85:* 305–6; and Gerrit Smith, *84:* 87

CALIFORNIA: Mazzini supported by Italians in, *62:* xliv, xlv; *63:* 272. *See also Pensiero e Azione; Roma del Popolo*

Canada: rumors of American invasion of, *81:* 230

Carbines: Mazzini wishes to buy, *26:* 79–80; *33:* 107; needs funds for, *26:* 80; insists on purchase of, *26:* 94; tries to buy, *Appendix 2:* 294–95; Alberto Mario doubts performance of, *Appendix 6:* 10–11. *See also* Arms

Carrel, Armand: advocates American Federalism for Italy, *77:* 147–48

Cass, Lewis, Jr.: disappoints Mazzini, *42:* 17; to be invited to clear Mazzini's name, *44:* 167; denies giving a passport to Mazzini, *57:* 116–17; asked to give American passports to Mazzini and others, *Appendix 6:* 543–44

Castiglia, Gaetano: deported to America, *12:* 169

Cavaleri, E.: supports Jessie W. Mario, *62:* 167–70

Charles and Jane: captured by Neapolitan cruiser, *68 :* 77

Charleston, South Carolina: Young Italy chapter founded in, *20:* 104

Christian Alliance: secret accord with, *23:* 269–71; and Lyman Beecher, *23:* 269; plans for propaganda with, *24:* 10; publicly established, *24:* 142, 153, 321; hopes of aid from, *24:* 233; *25:* 299–300; documents from, mailed to Paris, *24:* 237; errors in manifesto of, *24:* 239; promises help, *24:* 348–49; relations between Young Italy and, *28:* 177; will support revolution in Italy, *28:* 213; *Appendix 2:* 298; review of pamphlet of, *31:* 85–89; mentioned, *40:* 289; *52:* 147–48. *See also* Bargnani, Alessandro; Bargnani, Gaetano; MacMullen, John; Bible societies

Civil War: Mazzini opposes Garibaldi's participation in, *71:* 382–83, 393–94; *72:* 18, 30, 39; *Appendix 6:* 195; English hostility to the Union during, *72:* 193; Mazzini opposes

of, *30:* 321; Mazzini asks C. A. Biggs her opinion of, *33:* 298; ideas of, cannot inspire common man, *34:* 103; idealism of, *34:* 111; Mazzini receives a book by, *57:* 161; system of education of, *60:* 253; called an "idiot" by Mazzini, *70:* 245; to be invited to write for *People's Journal, Appendix, 6:* 516; Mazzini expects to see the opinion of, on his work, *Appendix 6:* 531

England: tense relations between America and, *20:* 110, 117; *28:* 218; *Appendix 5:* 105; American hostility to, *80:* 140, 178; understanding on America between France and, *80:* 339

Europe: Holy Alliance of the peoples of America and, *38:* 218, 219; recognition of revolutionary governments in, *47:* 258; sympathy for revolutionists of, *47:* 216; *49:* 279–80, 316–18, 340–41; *50:* 238; *51:* 33, 51, 165, 319

European Democracy: organization in America of, *44:* 64–65

Evening Post: sympathetic to Young Italy, *23:* 141

Exile to America: of Mazzini, *45:* 173; of Germans, *12:* 329, 375; of Italians, *44:* 39; of Poles, *34:* 61. *See also* Deportation

FAY, Theodore S. *See* Fey

Federal system: suited to America but not to Italy, *3:* 288–92; *25:* 262–63; *51:* 39–40; *77:* 47–48; *93:* 100; arguments in favor of, *3:* 265

Federalism: considered "doctrinaire," *3:* 266; tends to centralization *3:* 270–71; *85:* 335; opposed for Italy, *3:* 277–78; *10:* 151; *85:* 334–36; proposed for Italy by Angeloni, *14:* 251–52; *22:* 98; proposed by Carrel, *77:* 147–48; desired by Mazzini for Europe, *4:* 41–42; *13:* 181, 282; danger of doctrine of secession in, *25:* 261–62; in Italy, *53:* 259–60; Italian imitation of American, *62:* 275

Federalists, *3:* 261

Fey [Theodore S. Fay]: declares he will protect Mazzini, *53:* 129–30

Filopanti, Quirico: urged to organize Democrazia Europea in America,

44: 64; member of Committee for Associazione Nazionale, *44:* 77; urged to refute slander on Mazzini, *44:* 167

Fondo Nazionale: aid for, expected from New York, *32:* 298; drive for, urged on Foresti, *Appendix 3:* 41, 338

Forbes, Hugh: mission of, *42:* 95–96, 104, 112; is heard from, *42:* 261; sends report to Mazzini, *45:* 310; should remain in America, Mazzini thinks, *47:* 164; mentioned *44:* 168; *45:* 312

Foresti, Eleuterio F.: letters to, *33:* 79–82, 105–7, 226–31; *35:* 42–44; *42:* 14–18, 93–96, 261; *44:* 27–28, 62–69, 164–68; *45:* 59–62, 310–12; *47:* 137, 150, 161–64, 261–62, 306–7, 375; *53:* 126–27, 297–99; *56:* 111–12; *Appendix 3:* 41–42, 337–39; *Appendix 4:* 122; founds Young Italy in America, *20:* 105; President of Young Italy in America, *20:* 104, 262; *23:* 96; patriotic in spite of misfortunes, *20:* 309; *31:* 303–6; concerned over Mazzini's silence, *23:* 304–5; director of New York free school for poor Italians, *24:* 26; *77:* 272; expected in Paris, *24:* 193; in London, *24:* 244, 260–61; leaves for New York, *24:* 287; hears from Mazzini, *26:* 26, 56; receives pamphlet on Bandiera brothers, *27:* 134; *28:* 57; American collector for war chest funds, *28:* 59, 94, 302; receives copy of *Italy, Austria, and the Papal States, 28:* 148; recommends MacMullen to Lamberti, *28:* 203; contacts of, with South America, *33:* 82; representative of Roman Triumvirate in America, *40:* 250–51; reorganizes Italian patriotic associations in America, *42:* 17; *44:* 64; member of Committee of Associazione Nazionale, *44:* 77; receives bonds of National Loan, *44:* 164–66; *47:* 161; requested to cooperate with Lemmi, *47:* 104; recommended to Kossuth, *53:* 298; not heard from, *56:* 111; no longer a revolutionist, *57:* 57; introduces Coleman to Mazzini, *Appendix 3:* 41–42; mentioned, *20:* 371; *33:* 53

than in America, *32:* 221; inevitable in the future but different from the American, *77:* 310

Rescoflow, Otto: brings to Garibaldi funds subscribed in New York, *70:* 363–64

Richmond, Viginia: Young Italy chapter established in, by Carlo Bassini, *20:* 104

Roba di Roma. See Story, William W.

Roberti, Luigi: founds Young Italy chapter in New Haven, Conn., *20:* 104; Mazzini inquires about, *44:* 167

Roma del Popolo: mailed to San Francisco, *90:* 278

Rudio [unidentified Italian]: wishes to join Union army, *76:* 194–95, 320

Ruge, Arnold: writes against Mazzini in German language papers in America, *70:* 287

Russell, Thomas: copy of manifesto of National Italian Association mailed to, *44:* 98–99; secretary of Boston committee of Universal Republican Alliance, *84:* 80

SALINAS, Cristoforo: founds Young Italy chapter in Charleston, S.C., *20:* 104; Mazzini inquires about, *44:* 167

Sanders, George N.: letter to, *Appendix 5:* 219–20; gives an American passport to A. Saffi, *52:* 16; Mazzini can obtain an American passport from, *52:* 111; Jessie W. Mario has not met, *63:* 25, 29–30; not influential with Buchanan, *Appendix 5:* 194–95; advised to keep in touch with Avezzana and Ancarani, *Appendix 5:* 220

San Francisco, California: copy of Mazzini's *Parole* mailed to Mangini in, *65:* 374; copies of *Pensiero e Azione* mailed to Mangini in, *67:* 27; copies of *Roma del Popolo* mailed to Agostini in, *90:* 278

Sanguinetti [unidentified Genoese]: returns from New York, *15:* 299

Sartorio, Emanuele: teacher at the New York free school for poor Italians, *24:* 26

Schurz, Carl: letter to, *48:* 109–10; to be requested to deliver a message to Lincoln, *72:* 278–79

Secchi de Casali, G. F.: editor of Italian paper in New York, *44:* 210

Sedgwick, Katharine M.: mentions Mazzini and Young Italy in her *Letters from Abroad, 20:* 344–45, 350

Seward, William H.: reprimands Cushman, consul at Rome, *87:* 29–30

Siegel. *See* Bruzzesi, G.

Sismondi, Jean Charles de: on slavery in America, *17:* 244, 249

Slavery: in America, *3:* 277; *69:* 73; support of, by American republicans deplored, *6:* 106; Sismondi on, *17:* 244, 249; Mazzini opposed to, *53:* 342; called a blot on American institutions, *66:* 86; called a negation of God, *78:* 11; Mazzini interested in emancipated Negroes, *91:* 343

—Abolition of: supporters of, persecuted in America, *14:* 291; Marcus and Rebecca Spring in favor of, *30:* 321; letter in favor of, *52:* 175–77; reaction to letter on, *52:* 222–23; in Cuba, and American reaction, *62:* 36; British workers in favor of, *73:* 199–201; and the struggle of European liberals, *75:* 239–40; *76:* 33–34; a duty to God and Humanity, *80:* 127; result of political, not religious, crusade, *86:* 256. *See also* Brown, John; Garrison, William L.; *Concerning the Negro Question in America;* Kossuth, Louis; Mario, Jessie W.; *Prayer to God for the planters by an exile;* Remond, Sarah

Smith, Gerrit: letters to, *82:* 288–92; *84:* 73–75, 226–27; considered a wealthy, influential friend, *84:* 80–81; Bulewski fails with, *84:* 87; contributes five hundred dollars, *84:* 226

Society of Friends of Italy: to be founded in America, *45:* 311; organization of, urged on Foresti, *Appendix 4:* 122, to be initiated by Lemmi, *47:* 105

Soulé, Pierre: letter to, *Appendix 5:* 51–54; meets Mazzini, *49:* 317; expelled from France, *51:* 320; Mazzini expects a reply from, *53:* 259; Mazzini must see, *53:* 300; believed to hold funds to subsidize

REFERENCES AND NOTES

The following references are to books, articles, pamphlets, and newspaper items which the author found useful in the preparation of this monograph. This list is not intended to be a complete bibliography on Mazzini or on Mazzini's relations with the United States.

All references to Mazzini's writings are to the 100 volume *edizione nazionale*, *Scritti editi ed inediti* (Imola: Galeati, 1905–43).

"Address from the Democrats of England to the Democrats of the United States," Boston *Liberator* (June 24, 1853).

Address to the Friends of the Republican principles in America from the Friends of those principles in Europe with response thereto. New York, [1866].

Adresses of the Rev. L. Bacon, D.D., and Rev. Edward N. Kirk at the annual meeting of the Christian Alliance held in New York, May 8, 1845, with the Address of the Society and the Bull of the Pope against it. New York: S. W. Benedict, 1845.

Aldens, W. L. "Mazzini's Last Manifesto," *The Galaxy*, III (1867), 484–92.

Annual Report of the American and Foreign Christian Union. New York, 1853.

Anthony, Katharine. *Margaret Fuller.* New York: Harcourt, Brace & Howe, 1920.

Bell, Margaret. *Margaret Fuller.* New York: Boni, 1930.

Benedetti, Anna. "Mazzini e Margherita Fuller," *Nuova Antologia*, CCLXXVII (16 genn., 1918), 166–180.

Blind, Karl. "Personal Recollections about Garibaldi," *Frazer's Magazine*, CVI (1882), 236–54, 394–404.

Byron, George Gordon. *The Works of Lord Byron with his Letters and Journals, and his life.* Ed. Thomas Moore. vol. V. London: Murray, 1833.

Capobianco, Giuseppe L. "Il messaggio integrale di Abramo Lincoln a Macedonio Melloni," *Rassegna Storica del Risorgimento*, XVIII (1931), 458–67.

Carrel, Armand. *Oevres.* Vol. I. Paris: Chamerot, 1857.

Casanova, Eugenio. "A proposito della lettera di Abramo Lincoln a Macedonio Melloni," *Rassegna Storica del Risorgimento*, XVIII (1931), i–viii.

Codignola, Arturo. *La Giovinezza di G. Mazzini.* Firenze, 1926.

Colombo, Adolfo. "A proposito d'una lettera inedita di Giuseppe Mazzini al Sig. Soulé, ambasciatore degli Stati Uniti a Madrid," *Rassegna Storica del Risorgimento*, XIX (1932), 7–19.

Conway, Moncure D. *Mazzini: a discourse given in South Place chapel, Finsbury, March 17, 1872.* London: Printed by the author, 1872.

——. *Autobiography: Memories and Experiences.* 2 vols. New York: Houghton Mifflin Co., 1904.

Curti, Merle E. "Young America," *American Historical Review*, XXXII (Oct. 1926), 34–54.

——. "George N. Sanders—American Patriot of the Fifties," *South Atlantic Quarterly*, XXVII (1928), 79–87.

Detti, Emma. *Margaret Fuller-Ossoli e i suoi corrispondenti.* Firenze: Le Monnier, 1942.

Feraboli, Elsa. "Il primo esilio di Garibaldi in America," *Rassegna Storica del Risorgimento*, XIX (1932), 247–82.

Forbes, Hugh. *Four Lectures upon Recent Events in Italy Delivered in New York University.* New York: Fanshaw, 1851.

Franchi, Bruno. *Mazzini e Kossuth nei rapporti segreti della polizia austriaca in Dalmazia.* Zara: "San Marco" di G. Manni, 1938.

Frothingham, Octavius B. *Gerrit Smith.* New York: Putnam, 1878.

Fuller, Margaret S. "To a daughter of Italy," *The People's Journal*, IV (1847), 327–28.

——. *Memoirs.* Boston: Roberts Bros., 1881.

——. *At home and Abroad.* Boston: Roberts Bros., 1895.

——. *The Writings of Margaret Fuller.* ed. Mason Wade. New York: Viking Press, 1941.

Galimberti, Alice. "Giuseppe Mazzini nel pensiero inglese," *Nuova Antologia*, CCLXXXVI (1 luglio, 1919), 41–58.

Galpin, W. F. "Letters Concerning the 'Universal Republic,'" *American Historical Review*, XXXIV (1929), 779–86.

Garrison, William L. *Joseph Mazzini, his Life, Writings, and Political Principles.* New York: Hurd and Houghton, 1872.

Gay, Harry H. "Lincoln's Offer of a Command to Garibaldi," *Century Magazine*, LXXV (1907), 63–74.

——. *Scritti sul Risorgimento.* Roma: Rassegna Italiana, 1937.

Goggio, Emilio. "Cooper's Bravo in Italy," *Romanic Review*, XX (1929), 222–30.

——. "First Personal Contacts between American and Italian Leaders of Thought," *Romanic Review*, XXVII (1936), 1–8.

H., C. S. "Italian School, Greville-Street," *The People's Journal*, III (1847), Appendix, pp. 5–6.

Haney, John L. "Of the people, by the people, for the people," *Proceedings of the American Philosophical Society*, LXXXXVIII (1944), 359–67.

Harring, P. H. *Mémoirs sur la "Jeune Italie" et sur les derniers événements de Savoie.* Paris: Dérivaux, 1834.

Hinkley, Edyth. *Mazzini.* London: Allen & Unwin, 1924.

Hoeing W. "Letters of Mazzini to W. J. Linton," *Journal of Modern History*, V (1933), 55–68.

Italian Propagandism. New York: American and Foreign Christian Union, 1850.

"Italy and the Christian Alliance," [unsigned review of *Il Protestantesimo e la Regola di Fede*, per Giovanni Perrone. Roma: Civiltà Cattolica, 1853]

Brownson's Quarterly Review, XII (1855), 355–93.

Kastner, Eugenio. *Mazzini e Kossuth*. Firenze: Le Monnier, 1929.

King, Bolton. *Mazzini*. London: J. M. Dent, 1903.

Kossuth, Louis. *Selected Speeches*. Condensed and abridged by Francis W. Newman. London: Trubner & Co., 1853.

La Piana, Angelina. *La cultura americana e l'Italia*. Torino: Enaudi, 1938.

Librino, E. "Un rapporto diplomatico su Pietro Soulé," *Rassegna Storica del Risorgimento*, XIX (1932), 20–23.

Luzio, Alessandro. *Giuseppe Mazzini, Carbonaro*. Torino: Bocca, 1920.

McMaster, John B. *A History of the People of the United States*. vol. VII. New York: Appleton, 1910.

Mario, Jessie W. *Della vita di Giuseppe Mazzini*. Milano: Sonzogno, 1886.

Marraro, Howard R. *American Opinion on the Unification of Italy*. New York: Columbia University Press, 1932.

Mazzini, Giuseppe. "Mazzini on American Slavery," Boston *Liberator* (April 22, 1859).

———. "The Republican Alliance," *Atlantic Monthly*, XIX (1867), 235–45.

"Mazzini and Kossuth," Boston *Liberator* (July 30, 1852).

"Mazzini on American Slavery," Boston *Liberator* (Sept. 2, 1853).

Menghini, Mario. "Luigi Kossuth nel suo carteggio con Giuseppe Mazzini," *Rassegna Storica del Risorgimento*, VIII (1921) 1–171.

Morelli, Emilia. *Mazzini in Inghilterra*. Firenze: Le Monnier, 1938.

Nicolai, J. G. "Lincoln's Gettysburg Address," *Century Magazine*, XXV (1894), 596–608.

Nobécourt, René G. *La vie d'Armand Carrel*. Paris: Gallimard, 1930.

"The Papal Conspiracy Exposed," [unsigned review of *The Papal Conspiracy Exposed and Protestantism defended in the Light of Reason, History and Scriptures*, by Edward Beecher, D. D. Boston, 1855] *Brownson's Quarterly Review*, XII (1855), 246–70.

Parker, George F. "The Possible Origin of a Lincoln Phrase," *Review of Reviews*, XXIII (1901), 196.

Peterson, R. M. "Echoes of the Italian Risorgimento in Contemporaneous American Writers," *PMLA*, XLVII (1932), 220–40.

Prezzolini, Giuseppe. *Come gli Americani scoprirono l'Italia*. Milano: Treves, 1933.

Proceedings, Speeches, . . . at the Dinner given to Louis Kossuth at the National Hotel, Washington, Jan. 7, 1852. Washington: Printed at the Globe office, 1852.

Protocollo della Giovine Italia. Imola: Galeati, 1916–22.

Questions and Answers in Regard to the American and Foreign Christian Union. New York, 1849.

Report of the Special Committee appointed by the Common Council of the City of New York to make arrangements for the Reception of Gov. Louis Kossuth, the distinguished Hungarian patriot. New York: Published by order of the Common Council, 1852.

"The Revolutionary Secret Societies of Modern Italy," *United States Magazine and Democratic Review*, New Series, IX (1841), 260–76.

Rhodes, James F. *History of the United States*. 9 Vols. New York: Macmillan, new ed., 1928.

Rinaldi, Evelina. "Giuseppe Mazzini e gli Stati Uniti d'America," *Rassegna Storica del Risorgimento*, XIX (1932), 428–33.

Rostenberg, L. "Margaret Fuller's Roman Diary," *Journal of Modern History*, XII (1940), 209–20.

———. "Mazzini to Margaret Fuller," *American Historical Review*, XLVII (1941), 73–80.

Salvatorelli, Luigi. *Il pensiero politico italiano dal 1700 al 1870*. Torino: Enaudi, 2nd ed., 1941.

Salvemini, Gaetano. *Mazzini*. Firenze: La Voce, 4th ed., 1925.

Sanders, George N. *Illustrated Catalogue of the Political correspondence of the late Hon. George N. Sanders, Confederate Commissioner to Europe during the Civil War*. New York: The American Art Association, 1914.

Schiavo, Giovanni. *The Italians in America before the Civil War*. New York: Vigo Press, 1934.

———. *Four Centuries of Italian American History*. New York: S. F. Vanni, 1952.

Schurz, Carl. *The Reminiscences of Carl Schurz*. 3 vols. New York: McClure, 1907–8.

Sedgwick, Catherine M. *Letters from Abroad to Kindred at Home*. New York: Harpers & Bros., 1841.

Smith, Gerrit. "Gerrit Smith to Frederick Douglass," Boston *Liberator* (June 18, 1852).

Stafford, John. *The Literary Criticism of Young America*. Berkeley: University of California Press, 1952.

Stern, Madeleine B. *The Life of Margaret Fuller*. New York: E. P. Dutton, 1942.

Stillman, William J. *The Autobiography of a Journalist*. Boston: Houghton, Mifflin & Co., 1901.

Stock, Leo F. "An American Consul Joins the Papal Zouaves," *Catholic World*, CXXXII (1930), 145–50.

———. *United States Ministers to the Papal States*. Washington, D.C.: Catholic University Press, 1933.

———. *Consular Relations between the United States and the Papal States*. Washington, D.C.: American Catholic Historical Assn., 1945.

Tchernoff, J. *Le parti républicain sous la Monarchie de Juillet*. Paris: Pedone, 1905.

Thayer, William R. *The Dawn of Italian Independence*. Boston: Houghton, Mifflin & Co., 1892.

Trevelyan, George M. *Garibaldi's Defense of the Roman Republic*. London: Longmans, Green & Co., 1907.

———. *Garibaldi and the Making of Italy*. London: Longmans, Green & Co., 1912.

Visconti, Dante. *Le origini degli Stati Uniti d'America e l'Italia*. Padova: Cedam, 1940.

Wade, Mason. *Margaret Fuller: Whetstone of Genius*. New York: The Viking Press, 1940.

Weik, Jesse. "Lincoln's Gettysburg Address," *The Outlook*, CIV, (1913), 572–74.

Weill, Georges. *Histoire du parti républicain en France de 1814 à 1870*. Paris: Alcan, 1900.

"Young Italy and her American Allies," *United States Catholic Magazine*, IV (1845), 540–42.

CHAPTER I

1. See Visconti, *Le origini degli Stati Uniti d'America e l'Italia.*
2. Rinaldi, *"Giuseppe Mazzini e gli Stati Uniti d'America,* pp. 428–29. While in Ravenna Byron wrote in his diary on January 29, 1821: "Met a company of the sect (a kind of Liberal Club) called the 'Americani' in the forest, all armed, and singing, with all their might, in Romagnuole— 'Sem tutti soldat' per la libertà' ('We are all soldiers for liberty'). They cheered me as I passed." And on February 20, 1821, he wrote: "The 'Americani' . . . give a dinner in *the Forest* . . . and have invited me, as one of the C[arbonar]i."—*The Works of Lord Byron with His Letters and Journals, and His Life,* by Thomas Moore (London, 1833), V, 92, 105.
3. Mazzini, *Scritti editi ed inediti,* I, 40. Hereinafter references to the works are given in the text where they occur. The italized numerals indicate the volume, the numerals in roman type the page or pages.
4. Goggio, "Cooper's *Bravo* in Italy," pp. 222–30.
5. See Index of Americana, Appendix C.
6. Salvemini, *Mazzini,* pp. 15, 154; Salvatorelli, *Il pensiero politico italiano,* p. 229.
7. Weill, *Histoire du parti républicain en France,* Chapters 2, 3, and 4. See also Tchernoff, *Le parti républicain.*
8. Weill, *Histoire du parti républicain en France,* p. 43.
9. Tchernoff, *Le parti républicain,* p. 137.
10. *Ibid.,* p. 385.
11. Weill, *Histoire du parti républicain en France,* p. 52.
12. *Ibid.,* pp. 38, 258.
13. Salvatorelli, *Il pensiero politico italiano,* pp. 339–69.
14. Conway, *Autobiography,* II, 62.

15. Marraro, *American Opinion,* pp. 165–85.

CHAPTER II

1. *Protocollo della Giovine Italia,* I, 62.
2. Feraboli, "Il primo esilio di Garibaldi in America," p. 254. Garibaldi obtained letters of marque and reprisal from Benito Gonzales, leader of the republicans of Rio Grande. See Mario, *Della vita di Giuseppe Mazzini,* p. 264, for the first "action" of the *Mazzini.*
3. *Protocollo della Giovine Italia,* I, 118.
4. *Ibid.,* III, 16.
5. *Ibid.,* p. 66.
6. *Ibid.,* p. 16.
7. *Ibid.,* I, 113.
8. "The Revolutionary Secret Societies of Modern Italy," pp. 260–76.
9. *Ibid.,* pp. 270–71.
10. Sedgwick, *Letters from Abroad,* II, 121–24.
11. New Orleans *Daily Picayune,* November 5, 6, 1846; *L'Abeille de la Nouvelle Orléans,* November 5, 6, 1846; *Le Courrier de la Louisiane,* November 5, 6, 1846; *The Daily Tropic,* November 4, 5, 6, 1846; *The Daily Delta,* November 5, 6, 1846.

CHAPTER III

1. McMaster, *A History of the People of the United States,* VII, 371. The Leopold Foundation or Leopoldine Society was founded in Vienna in 1829 to aid Catholic missions in North America. It was patterned after the French Society for the Propagation of the Faith founded in Lyons in 1822, and was named after Leopoldina, a favorite daughter of Francis I of Austria and wife of Pedro I of Brazil.
2. The Reverend Edward Beecher, D.D., a son of Lyman Beecher, president of the Christian Alliance, and

himself a member of the Board of Councilors of that Body, expounded this theory of Papal conspiracy in a book entitled *The Papal Conspiracy Exposed*. An unsigned review of the book in *Brownson's Quarterly Review* countered with an accusation of a Protestant conspiracy against Catholicism in a reference to the alliance with Mazzini: "Everybody knows that Protestants express their determination to exterminate Catholicity, not in our country only, but in all countries. To this end they have formed and sustained alliances and associations, in conjunction with acknowledged conspirators, for the purpose of revolutionizing every Catholic state in Europe, in the hope that, by revolutionizing the state in the sense of Red Republicanism, they will put an end to the Papacy, to Catholicity."—"The Papal Conspiracy Exposed," p. 249.

3. Prezzolini, *Come gli Americani scoprirono l'Italia*, p. 262.

4. *Protocollo della Giovine Italia*, III, 16.

5. *Ibid.*, II, 41.

6. *Addresses of the Rev. L. Bacon and Rev. Edward N. Kirk*, pp. 3–6.

7. *Ibid.*, pp. 32–35.

8. *Ibid.*, pp. 44–46.

9. *Ibid.*, p. 7.

10. "Young Italy and Her American Allies," pp. 540–42.

11. "Italy and the Christian Alliance," pp. 355–93.

12. Reprinted in "Young Italy and Her American Allies," p. 541.

13. *Addresses of the Rev. L. Bacon and Rev. Edward N. Kirk*, p. 7.

14. See *Protocollo della Giovine Italia*, Vols. III and IV.

15. *National Protestant Magazine*, III (1846), 200–201.

16. "Italy and the Christian Alliance," p. 362.

17. Salvemini, *Mazzini*, pp. 203–4.

18. See the *New York Tribune*, February 24, 1851.

19. See Forbes, *Four Lectures*. No biographical sketch of this interesting adventurer has been located. From scattered references we gather the following facts about his American career. In 1851 his financial condition was so precarious that he contemplated returning to England, an eventuality that alarmed Mazzini.—*Scritti*, XLVII, 164. He must have remained in America, because in 1853 Garibaldi mentioned him as being in New York.—Gay, *Scritti sul Risorgimento*, p. 212. In 1856 he appeared before the Mayor of New York to plead the case of destitute Italian refugees from the Papal states.—Marraro, *American Opinion*, p.181. The following year he stopped at Peterboro to visit Gerrit Smith who provided him with the means to join John Brown in Kansas.—Frothingham, *Gerrit Smith*, p. 237. He served under John Brown as drill master, then followed him back east, but refused to go along with him to the Harper's Ferry expedition, which he caused to be delayed for several months by revealing Brown's plan to Senators Brown and Seward. —Rhodes, *History of the United States*, II, 388–89. He was back in Italy in 1860 when he joined Garibaldi in Sicily. He suggested to Garibaldi the formation of an English Volunteer Brigade, but when, against the wiser counsel of other Englishmen, the Brigade was organized, he was not given its command, and was left behind in Sicily as Governor of the Milazzo Castle.—Trevelyan, *Garibaldi and the Making of Italy*, p. 98. For his part in Garibaldi's retreat after the fall of the Roman republic in 1849, see Trevelyan, *Garibaldi's Defense of the Roman Republic*, pp. 252–99.

20. *Questions and Answers in Regard to the American and Foreign Christian Union.*

21. Forbes, *Four Lectures*, p. 110.

22. *Ibid.*, p. 105.

23. *Annual Report of the American and Foreign Christian Union*, 1953, pp. 52–53.

24. *Protocollo della Giovine Italia*, III, 324, 325. John L. O'Sullivan, who visited Lamberti in Paris on October 27, 1845, was the editor and co-founder of the *New York Morning News*. On February 6, 1857, he called on Mazzini, who evidently had not met him before, because he referred to him as "Sullivan," "American consul or ambassador in Portugal." —*Scritti*, LVII, 302. He was the American ambassador to Portugal from 1854 to 1858.

CHAPTER IV

1. Wade, *Margaret Fuller*, p. 185.

2. Anthony, *Margaret Fuller*, pp. 178–79.

3. Wade, *Margaret Fuller*, p. 93.

4. Morelli, *Mazzini in Inghilterra*, p. 38.

5. Fuller, *At Home and Abroad*, p. 181.

6. Harring, *Mémoirs sur la "Jeune Italie."*

7. Stern, *Life of Margaret Fuller*, pp. 360–61.

8. Fuller, *Memoirs*, II, 173, 187.

9. *Ibid.*, pp. 187–88.

10. C. S. H., "Italian School, Greville-Street," pp. 5–6.

11. Fuller, *At Home and Abroad*, pp. 182–83.

12. Fuller, *Writings*, p. 581.

13. *Protocollo della Giovine Italia*, IV, 197.

14. *Ibid.*, V, 3.

15. *Ibid.*, IV, 213.

16. *Ibid.*, V, 7.

17. Fuller, *At Home and Abroad*, p. 217.

18. Detti, *Margaret Fuller-Ossoli*, pp. 348–49.

19. Fuller, "To a Daughter of Italy," pp. 327–28.

20. Fuller, *At Home and Abroad*, p. 320.

21. Fuller, *Writings*, pp. 581–82.

22. Fuller, *Memoirs*, II, 262–63.

23. Fuller, *At Home and Abroad*, p. 439.

24. Marraro, *American Opinion*, pp. 165–66.

25. Fuller, *Memoirs*, II, 268.

26. *Ibid.*, p. 350; Fuller, *At Home and Abroad*, pp. 447, 451.

27. Mario, *Della vita di Mazzini*, p. 348.

28. Wade, *Margaret Fuller*, p. 281.

29. *Ibid.*, pp. 276–77.

30. *Ibid.*, p. 278.

31. Fuller, *At Home and Abroad*, p. 439.

CHAPTER V

1. Stock, *United States Ministers*, pp. 5–6. The request seems suggestive of a popular appeal of America, other indications of which are found at that time. The call of the American frigate *Princeton* at the Roman port of Civitavecchia in 1847 gave rise to rumors and speculations among which the one that the purpose of the call was "to sustain the cause of Pius IX against his foes," as the American vice-consul reported to Washington.—Stock, *Consular Relations*, p. 115. On January 1, 1848, the Milanese began a boycott of the tobacco monopoly, to deprive the Austrian Treasury of the considerable revenue derived from that source. A Prof. Cantoni, who wrote the manifesto, "cited the example of the fellow-citizens of Washington and Franklin, who had thrown overboard the taxed tea of 'avaricious England.'"—Thayer, *Dawn of Italian*

Independence, II, 102. On the evening of May 13, 1848, the police in Leghorn forbade a public demonstration in favor of Pius IX; in defiance of the order, the people paraded through the streets following an American flag and crying, "Long live the Republic!"—De Boni, *Così la penso*, quoted in Mazzini, *Scritti*, XXXII, 154–55.

2. Stock, *Consular Relations*, p. 170.
3. *Ibid.*, p. 171.
4. *Ibid.*, p. 174.
5. Stock, *United States Ministers*, pp. 39–40.
6. *Ibid.*, pp. 44–45.
7. Marraro, *American Opinion*, p. 72.
8. *Ibid.*, pp. 91–92.
9. *Ibid.*, pp. 89–91.
10. Detti, *Margaret Fuller-Ossoli*, p. 340.
11. Marraro, *American Opinion*, p. 71.
12. Stock, *Consular Relations*, pp. 163–64. Even Cass' predecessor, Dr. Martin, noticed and reported on this British hostility to the revolutionary movement in Italy. "A struggle is now going on," he wrote to Buchanan on April 1, 1848, "perhaps a doubtful one, in which Rome takes a part, for the independence of Italy, which has the lively sympathies of France, but on which England is supposed to look with no friendly eye."—Stock, *United States Ministers*, p. 5.
13. Stock, *United States Ministers*, p. 52.
14. *Ibid.*, pp. 58–59.
15. Menghini, "Luigi Kossuth," p. 159.
16. Marraro, *American Opinion*, p. 174.
17. Stock, *Consular Relations*, p. 325.
18. *Ibid.*, pp. 325–34. See also Stock, "An American Consul Joins

the Papal Zouaves," pp. 145–50.

CHAPTER VI

1. Kastner, *Mazzini e Kossuth*, pp. 2–3.
2. *Ibid.*, p. 23.
3. *Ibid.*, p. 108.
4. *Ibid.*, pp. 140–63.
5. *Ibid.*, p. 27.
6. Rhodes, *History of the United States*, I, 223, 236. For a discussion of Kossuth's visit, see *Rhodes, ibid.*, pp. 231–43.
7. Menghini, "Luigi Kossuth," pp. 117–19.
8. *Report of the Special Committee for the Reception of Kossuth*, p. 104.
9. *Ibid.*, pp. 142, 144.
10. *Ibid.*, p. 616.
11. Kossuth, *Selected Speeches*, pp. 303, 306–9.
12. *Report of the Special Committee for the Reception of Kossuth*, p. 254.
13. *Ibid.*, pp. 481, 490.
14. *Ibid.*, pp. 695–700.
15. *Ibid.*, p. 426.
16. *Ibid.*, p. 560.
17. Menghini, "Luigi Kossuth," pp. 79–80.
18. *Ibid.*, pp. 87–88.
19. *Ibid.*, pp. 82–84.

CHAPTER VII

1. Curti, "Young America," p. 34.
2. Stillman, *Autobiography of a Journalist*, I, 143–44.
3. Rhodes, *History of the United States*, I, 416–19.
4. Menghini, "Luigi Kossuth," p. 165.
5. *Ibid.*, pp. 164–65.
6. King, *Mazzini*, p. 171.
7. Curti, "Young America," p. 48.
8. *New York Herald*, December 24, 1858.
9. Curti, "Young America," p. 41.

10. Menghini, "Luigi Kossuth," p. 84.

11. Curti, "Young America," p. 51.

12. *Ibid.*, pp. 45–46.

13. Colombo, "A proposito d'una lettera inedita di Giuseppe Mazzini," pp. 11–12.

14. *Ibid.*, p. 13.

15. Menghini, "Luigi Kossuth," pp. 159–61.

16. Librino, "Un rapporto diplomatico su Pietro Soulé," p. 23.

17. Rhodes, *History of the United States*, I, 547.

18. Sanders, *Illustrated Catalogue of the Political Correspondence of George Sanders*, Nos. 144–51.

CHAPTER VIII

1. Marraro, *American Opinion*, p. 209.

2. *Ibid.*, p. 210.

3. *Ibid.*, pp. 205–21.

4. *New York Herald*, December 2, 1858.

5. Marraro, *American Opinion*, p. 218.

6. *New York Herald*, December 2, 1858.

7. *New York Times*, December 9, 1858.

8. *New York Tribune*, December 16, 1858.

9. New York *Evening Post Semi-Weekly*, December 18, 1858.

10. *New York Tribune*, December 21, 1858.

11. *New York Herald*, December 2, 1858.

12. *Ibid.*

13. *New York Tribune*, December 2, 1858.

14. *New York Times*, December 9, 1858.

15. *Ibid.*, December 13, 1858.

16. *Ibid.*, December 15, 1858.

17. *Ibid.*, December 16, 1858.

18. *Ibid.*, December 18, 1858.

19. *Ibid.*

20. *New York Tribune*, February 2, 1859.

21. Marraro, *American Opinion*, pp. 178–80.

22. *New York Times*, January 10, 1859.

23. *Ibid.*, January 13, 1859.

24. *Ibid.*, January 14, 1859.

25. *Ibid.*, January 27, 1859.

26. *Ibid.*, January 1, 1859.

27. *Ibid.*, January 17, 1859.

28. *New York Tribune*, January 19, 1859.

29. *Ibid.*, February 4, 1859.

30. *New York Times*, February 16, 1859; Washington, D.C., *Weekly National Intelligencer*, February 19, 1859.

31. *Baltimore Sun*, March 10, 21, 1859.

32. New York *Evening Post Semi-Weekly*, December 25, 1859.

CHAPTER IX

1. The text of this abolitionist letter is not found either in Mazzini's *Scritti* or in the Boston *Liberator* of 1852 or 1853. Since it is not likely that Garrison would publish Mazzini's letter elsewhere than in his *Liberator*, and since Mazzini did later state that he had never been in private correspondence with Garrison (*Scritti*, LX, 379), the letter referred to may have been his adhesion to the "Address from the Democrats of England to the Democrats of the United States," published in the *Liberator* of June 24, 1853, over the signature of Mazzini's old friend, George Jacob Holyoake, and reportedly subscribed by 1857 other democrats of England. If this hypothesis is correct it is amusing to note that while the stand of the address displeased Kossuth and his

southern friends, the mildness of that stand was strongly criticized by extreme abolitionists like Garrison in America and Linton in England, and led to a controversy conducted in the columns of the *Liberator* between Garrison and Linton on one side and Holyoake and Harriet Martineau on the other. Another possibility is that the quarrel between Kossuth and Mazzini took place because of an item published in the *Liberator* of September 2, 1853, under the title "Mazzini on American Slavery," which, though not given as correspondence from Mazzini, may have been based on some letter of his not otherwise published. Since there is a reference to Kossuth, one can understand how Kossuth could well be annoyed by its publication. It reads as follows:

"The interests of Humanity are one. The interests of Freedom are one. Whatever pertains to the welfare of one portion of the race pertains to all. God hath made of one blood all nations of men. God hath joined the fate of all so together that one portion of the race cannot suffer, but all suffer with it. Hence no true friend of Liberty can be other than a hater of all slavery. And hence, every blow struck for freedom, though in the uttermost parts of the earth, is a blow on the head of every form of tyranny over the soul of man, no matter what his complexion or his race. The brave word spoken for Hungarian or Italian liberty, is a word, too, for American Liberty, and against American Slavery. So the advocates of American slavery know and feel. And hence the coldness and opposition with which they meet the champions of Freedom in other lands. This is the solution of Southern dislike to Kossuth, who made the mistake of trying to ignore

a fact which blocked his path at every step during his sojourn in America. His noble compatriot, Mazzini, the prophet-hero of Italy, understands this principle better."

2. Boston *Liberator*, July 21, 1854, where are also published Mazzini's letter and a number of comments from other papers.

3. *Ibid.*

4. Sanders, *Illustrated Catalogue of the Political Correspondence of George Sanders*, No. 71. The letter was obviously misdated March 14, 1854, since it discusses Kossuth's letter dated June 3, 1854.

5. See "Gerrit Smith to Frederick Douglass," Boston *Liberator*, June 18, 1852; "Mazzini and Kossuth," *ibid.*, July 30, 1852; "Mazzini on American Slavery," *ibid.*, September 2, 1853.

6. Boston *Liberator*, January 7, 1853.

7. *Ibid.*, April 22, 1859.

8. Conway, *Autobiography*, I, 422; II, 31.

9. Garrison, *Joseph Mazzini*, Intro. p. vii.

10. Conway, *Autobiography*, II, 58, 65, 67.

11. Blind, "Personal Recollections about Garibaldi," p. 244.

12. Gay, "Lincoln's offer of a Command to Garibaldi," pp. 63–74; Gay, *Scritti sul Risorgimento*, pp. 233–49.

13. Capobianco, "Il messaggio integrale di Abramo Lincoln a Macedonio Melloni," p. 467. See also Casanova, "A proposito della lettera di Abramo Lincoln a Macedonio Melloni," pp. i–viii.

14. See Nicolai, "Lincoln's Gettysburg Address," pp. 606–8; Parker, "Possible Origin of a Lincoln Phrase," p. 196; Weik, "Lincoln's Gettysburg Address," pp. 572–74; Haney, "Of the people, by the

people, for the people," pp. 359–67.

15. Nobécourt, *La vie d'Armand Carrel*, p. 136. See also Carrel, *Œuvres*, I, xxxiv.

16. Kossuth, *Selected Speeches*, p. 185.

CHAPTER X

1. Conway, *Autobiography*, II, 62–63, 64.

2. *New York Tribune*, April 23, 1866.

3. *Ibid.*

4. *Boston Daily Advertiser*, June 19, 1866. This writer was unable to locate the English text of the response of the Boston committee. It was not published in the *Advertiser*, which carried the story of the organization of the committee and the text of the response of the New York committee.

5. *Address to the Friends of the Republican principles in America.* Published also in the *Boston Daily Advertiser*, June 20, 1866.

6. A facsimile of a subscription note in Mazzini, *Scritti*, LXXXVI, 52.

7. Gerrit Smith to Mazzini, November 14, 1851. Holograph copy in the Gerrit Smith-Miller Collection in Syracuse University Library. See Appendix A.

8. Boston *Liberator*, June 18, 1852.

9. Galpin, "Letters Concerning the 'Universal Republic,'" pp. 780–81.

10. For the English text, see Mazzini, "The Republican Alliance," pp. 235–45. An adverse criticism is found in Alden, "Mazzini's Last Manifesto," pp. 484–92.

11. Galpin, "Letters Concerning the 'Universal Republic'," pp. 785–86.

12. *Ibid.*, pp. 783–84.

CHAPTER XI

1. Salvemini, *Mazzini*, pp. 101–2.

INDEX

Pisacane, Carlo, 98, 107
Pius IX: popular enthusiasm for, 52,
    62; flees Rome, 57; tyranny of,
    110–11
Poe, Edgar Allan, 3
Polk, James K., 62
Pyat, Félix, 96

RASPAIL, François, 4
Raymond, Henry J., 110, 140
Remond, Sarah, 128
Roberti, Luigi, 19
Robespierre, Maximilien de, 6
Ronchi, Ambrogio, 93
Rossi, Pellegrino, 56
Rothwell, Richard, 73
Ruffini, Agostino, 15
Ruffini, Giovanni, 15
Ruge, Arnold, 77, 79
Russell, Thomas, 45, 145
Russia: contrasted with America,
    83–84

SAFFI, Aurelio, 76, 95, 96
Saint-Just, Louis de, 6
Salazar di Promanengo, Fulvia, 134
Salinas, Cristoforo, 19
Sand, George, 52, 53
Sanders, George N.: leader of Young
    America, 91; consul at London,
    95; and European liberals, 95–98;
    and European conservatives, 98,
    99; and Jessie White Mario, 110;
    Mazzini disappointed in, 121; and
    Kossuth, 126; Mazzini's letters to,
    157–58; mentioned, 124
Sanford, H. S., 131
Sartorio, Emanuele, 25
Schurz, Carl, 130, 131
Sedgwick, Catherine Maria, 23
Seward, William H.: reprimands
    E. D. Cushman, 73–74
Sismondi, Jean Charles de, 4, 8, 23
Smith, Gerrit: abolitionism of, 128;
    and the Universal Republican
    Alliance, 140, 144, 145, 146, 147;
    letter to Mazzini, 155
Soulé, Pierre: and Young America,

92, 95; and Mazzini, 93–94, 102;
    L. Mossi on, 100; and Ostend
    Manifesto, 101; Mazzini's letter to,
    102–104; mentioned, 28, 124
Spring, Marcus: meets G. Lamberti,
    52; Margaret Fuller's letter to, 57–
    58; contribution of, to National
    Loan, 78
Spring, Marcus and Rebecca: and
    Margaret Fuller, 49; and the Weld
    school, 120; abolitionism of, 124,
    128
Stansbury, E. A., 140, 145
Sterns, G. L., 145
Stowe, Harriet Beecher, 3

TAYLOR, Clementia, 128, 129
Thompson, George, 124
Thompson, Th. Perronet, 124
Thoreau, Henry, David, 3
Tinelli, Luigi, 13
Trélat, Ulysse, 4

UNIVERSAL Republican Alliance:
    founded in America, 139–41; or-
    ganized in Italy, 147–48; men-
    tioned, 149

VIEUSSEUX, Giampietro, 8

WALMSLEY, Joshua, 96
Washington, George, 2, 6, 13, 82,
    105, 141
Weed, Thurlow, 140
Weld, Theodore D.: and Jessie
    White Mario, 120; Mazzini's letter
    to, 127–28, 158–59
Whitman, Walt, 3

YOUNG America: and the Demo-
    cratic Party, 91–92; and Mazzini,
    92–98; mentioned, 90, 149
Young Italy: founding of, 3; re-
    organization of, 16; in America,
    17–30; schools in London, Boston,
    and New York, 24–25; activity in
    New Orleans, 27–29; dissolved,
    29–30; mentioned 149